Quality of Care for
Oncologic Conditions and HIV

A Review of the Literature and Quality Indicators

Steven M. Asch • Eve A. Kerr • Eric G. Hamilton

Jennifer L. Reifel • Elizabeth A. McGlynn

Editors

RAND Health

Supported by the Agency for Healthcare Research and Quality

Principal funding for this report was provided by a cooperative agreement from the Agency for Healthcare Research and Quality.

ISBN: 0-8330-2920-7

Published 2000 by RAND
1700 Main Street, P.O. Box 2138, Santa Monica, CA 90407-2138
1200 South Hayes Street, Arlington, VA 22202-5050
RAND URL: http://www.rand.org/
To order RAND documents or to obtain additional information, contact Distribution Services: Telephone: (310) 451-7002;
Fax: (310) 451-6915; Internet: order@rand.org

PREFACE

This report is one of a series of volumes describing the QA Tools, a comprehensive, clinically based system for assessing care for children and adults. The quality indicators that comprise these Tools cover 46 clinical areas and all 4 functions of medicine—screening, diagnosis, treatment, and follow-up. The indicators also cover a variety of modes of providing care, including history, physical examination, laboratory study, medication, and other interventions and contacts.

Development of each indicator was based on a review of the literature. Each volume documents the literature on which the indicators were based, explains how the clinical areas and indicators were selected, and describes what is included in the overall system.

The QA Tools were developed with funding from public and private sponsors—the Health Care Financing Administration, the Agency for Healthcare Research and Quality, the California HealthCare Foundation, and the Robert Wood Johnson Foundation.

The other four volumes in this series are:

Quality of Care for General Medical Conditions: A Review of the Literature and Quality Indicators. Eve A. Kerr, Steven M. Asch, Eric G. Hamilton, and Elizabeth A. McGlynn, eds. MR-1280-AHRQ, 2000.

Quality of Care for Cardiopulmonary Conditions: A Review of the Literature and Quality Indicators. Eve A. Kerr, Steven M. Asch, Eric G. Hamilton, and Elizabeth A. McGlynn, eds. MR-1282-AHRQ, 2000.

Quality of Care for Children and Adolescents: A Review of Selected Clinical Conditions and Quality Indicators. Elizabeth A. McGlynn, Cheryl L. Damberg, Eve A. Kerr, and Mark A. Schuster, eds. MR-1283-HCFA, 2000.

Quality of Care for Women: A Review of Selected Clinical Conditions and Quality Indicators. Elizabeth A. McGlynn, Eve A. Kerr, Cheryl L. Damberg, and Steven M. Asch, eds. MR-1284-HCFA, 2000.

These volumes should be of interest to clinicians, health plans, insurers, and health services researchers. At the time of publication, the QA Tools system was undergoing testing in managed care plans, medical groups, and

selected communities. For more information about the QA Tools system, contact
RAND_Health@rand.org.

CONTENTS

TABLES

FIGURES

ACKNOWLEDGEMENTS

Funding for this work was provided by a Cooperative Agreement (No. 5U18HS09463-02), "Adult Global Quality Assessment Tool") from the Agency for Healthcare Research and Quality. We appreciate the continued and enthusiastic support of our project officer, Elinor Walker.

We are indebted to our expert panelists who gave generously of their time, knowledge and wisdom:

Lodovico Balducci, M.D. (Panel Chair)
Professor of Medicine and Program Leader
Senior Adult Oncology Program
Division of Medical Oncology and Hematology
H. Lee Moffitt Cancer Center & Research Institute
U.S.F. College of Medicine
Tampa, FL

Al B. Benson, III, M.D., F.A.C.P.
Professor of Medicine
Director, Clinical Investigations Program
Robert H. Lurie Cancer Center
Division of Hematology/Oncology
Northwestern University
Chicago, IL

Douglas W. Blayney, M.D., F.A.C.P.
Medical Director, Oncology Program
Robert and Beverly Lewis Family Cancer Care Center
Pomona Valley Hospital Medical Center
Pomona, CA

Paul F. Engstrom, M.D.
Senior Vice President, Population Science
Fox Chase Cancer Center
Philadelphia, PA

Howard I. Scher, M.D.
Associate Chairman, MSK Network
Chief, Genitourinary Oncology Service
Division of Solid Tumor Oncology
Department of Medicine
Memorial Sloan-Kettering Cancer Center
New York, NY

Barbara J. Turner, M.D., M.S.Ed., F.A.C.P.
Director, Division of Health Care Research
Center for Research in Medical Education and Health Care
Thomas Jefferson University
Philadelphia, PA

Jamie H. Von Roenn, M.D.
Associate Professor of Medicine
Northwestern University School of Medicine
Division of Hematology/Oncology
Northwestern University
Chicago, IL

James Lloyd Wade, III, M.D.
Director, Medical Oncology
Decatur Memorial Hospital
Cancer Care Specialists of Central Illinois
Decatur, IL

Neil Wenger, M.D.
Associate Director
Fellowship Program in Health Services Research
Associate Professor
UCLA Department of Medicine
Los Angeles, CA

Our thanks also go to the following experts who reviewed and provided consulatation on specific chapters:

Samuel Bozzette, M.D., Ph.D., RAND (HIV Disease)

Allen Gifford, M.D., University of California at San Diego (HIV Disease)

Allen McCutchan, M.D., University of California at San Diego (HIV Disease)

We are also greatly indebted to the following project staff whose contributions made this document possible: Kenneth Clark, Landon Donsbach, Sandy Geschwind, Kevin Heslin, Nicole Humphrey, Amy Kilbourne, and Tammy Majeski.

INTRODUCTION

Developing and implementing a valid system of quality assessment is essential for effective functioning of the health care system. Although a number of groups have produced quality assessment tools, these tools typically suffer from a variety of limitations. Information is obtained on only a few dimensions of quality, the tools rely exclusively on administrative data, they examine quality only for users of services rather than the population, or they fail to provide a scientific basis for the quality indicators.

Under funding from public and private sponsors, including the Health Care Financing Administration (HCFA), the Agency for Healthcare Research and Quality (AHRQ), the California HealthCare Foundation, and the Robert Wood Johnson Foundation (RWJ), RAND has developed and tested a comprehensive, clinically based system for assessing quality of care for children and adults. We call this system QA Tools.

In this introduction, we discuss how the clinical areas were selected, how the indicators were chosen, and what is included in the overall system. We then describe in detail how we developed the indicators for children and adolescents.

ADVANTAGES OF THE QA TOOLS SYSTEM

QA Tools is a comprehensive, clinically based system for assessing the quality of care for children and adults. The indicators cover 46 clinical areas and all four functions of medicine including screening, diagnosis, treatment, and follow-up. The indicators also cover a variety of modes of providing care, such as history, physical examination, laboratory study, medication, and other interventions and contacts. Initial development of indicators for each clinical area was based on a review of the literature.

The QA Tools system addresses many limitations of current quality assessment tools by offering the following:

- They are clinically detailed and require data typically found in medical records rather than just relying exclusively on data from administrative records.

1

- They examine quality for a population-based sample rather than for a more restricted sample of those who use care or have insurance.
- They document the scientific basis for developing and choosing the indicators.
- The QA Tools system is designed to target populations vulnerable to underutilization.
- Because of the comprehensiveness of the system, it is difficult for health care organizations to focus on a few indicators to increase their quality scores.
- QA Tools is a system that can be effective for both internal and external quality reviews. Health care organizations can use the system in order to improve the overall quality of the care provided.
- Because of the simple summary scores that will be produced, it will be an important tool for purchasers and consumers who are making choices about health care coverage and which provider to see.

Given its comprehensiveness, the QA Tools system contrasts with *leading indicators*, the most common approach to quality measurement in use today. Under the leading indicators approach, three to five specific quality measures are selected across a few domains (for example, rates of mammography screening, prevalence of the use of beta blockers among persons who have had a heart attack, and appropriateness of hysterectomy).

Leading indicators may work well for drawing general conclusions about quality when they correlate highly with other similar but unmeasured interventions and when repeated measurement and public reporting does not change the relationship of those indicators to the related interventions. However, to date no real evaluation of the utility of leading indicators in assessing health system performance has been done. We also do not know whether the selected indicators currently in use consistently represent other unmeasured practices.

By contrast, a comprehensive system can represent different dimensions of quality of care delivery by using a large number of measures applied to a population of interest and aggregated to produce index scores to draw conclusions about quality. A comprehensive system works well when evidence exists of variability within and between the diagnosis and management of different conditions and when the question being asked is framed at a high level (for instance, how well is the health system helping the population stay healthy, or how much of a problem does underuse present?).

In the 46 clinical areas they encompass, the QA Tools adequately represent scientific and expert judgment on what constitutes quality care. However, both the science and the practice of medicine continue to evolve. For the QA Tools to remain a valid tool for quality assessment over time, the scientific evidence in each area needs to be reviewed annually to determine if new evidence warrants modifying the indicators and/or clinical areas included in the system.

SELECTING CLINICAL AREAS FOR THE QA TOOLS

We reviewed Vital Statistics, the National Health Interview Survey, the National Hospital Discharge Survey, and the National Ambulatory Medical Care Survey to identify the leading causes of morbidity and mortality and the most common reasons for physician visits in the United States. We examined statistics for different age and gender groups in the population (0-1, 1-5, 6-11, 12-17, 18-50 [men and women], 50-64, 65-75, over 75).

We selected topics that reflected these different areas of importance (death, disability, utilization of services) and that covered preventive care as well as care for acute and chronic conditions. In addition, we consulted with a variety of experts to identify areas that are important to these various populations but that may be underrepresented in national data sets (for example, mental health problems). Finally, we sought to select enough clinical areas to represent a majority of the health care delivery system.

Table I.1 lists the 46 clinical areas included in the QA Tools system by population group; 20 include indicators for children and 36 for adults. The clinical areas, broadly defined, represent about 55 percent of the reasons for ambulatory care visits among children, 50 percent of the reasons for ambulatory care visits for the entire population, and 46 percent of the reasons for hospitalization among adults.

Note: Table I.1 reflects the clinical areas that were included in the system currently being tested. Several clinical areas (e.g., lung cancer, sickle cell disease) for which indicators were developed were not incorporated into the current tool due to budgetary constraints.

3

Table I.1

Clinical Areas in QA Tools System By Covered Population Group

Clinical Areas	Children	Adults
Acne	X	
Adolescent preventive services	X	
Adult screening and prevention		X
Alcohol dependence		X
Allergic rhinitis	X	
Asthma	X	X
Atrial fibrillation		X
Attention deficit/hyperactivity disorder	X	
Benign prostatic hyperplasia		X
Breast cancer		X
Cataracts		X
Cerebrovascular disease		X
Cervical cancer		X
Cesarean delivery	X	X
Chronic obstructive pulmonary disease		X
Colorectal cancer		X
Congestive heart failure		X
Coronary artery disease		X
Depression	X	X
Developmental screening	X	
Diabetes Mellitus	X	X
Diarrheal disease	X	
Family planning and contraception	X	X
Fever of unknown origin	X	
Headache		X
Hip fracture		X
Hormone replacement therapy		X
Human immunodeficiency virus		X
Hyperlipidemia		X
Hypertension		X
Immunizations	X	X
Low back pain		X
Orthopedic conditions		X
Osteoarthritis		X
Otitis media	X	
Pain management for cancer		X
Peptic ulcer disease & dyspepsia		X
Pneumonia		X
Prenatal care and delivery	X	X
Prostate cancer		X
Tuberculosis	X	X
Upper respiratory tract infections	X	
Urinary tract infections	X	X
Uterine bleeding and hysterectomy		X
Vaginitis and sexually transmitted diseases	X	X
Well child care	X	
Total number of clinical areas	**20**	**36**

SELECTING QUALITY INDICATORS

In this section, we describe the process by which indicators were chosen for inclusion in the QA Tools system. This process involved RAND staff drafting proposed indicators based on a review of the pertinent clinical literature and expert panel review of those indicators.

Literature Review

For each clinical area chosen, we reviewed the scientific literature for evidence that effective methods of prevention, screening, diagnosis, treatment, and follow-up existed (Kerr et al., 2000a; Kerr et al., 2000b; McGlynn et al., 2000a; McGlynn et al., 2000b). We explicitly examined the continuum of care in each clinical area. RAND staff drafted indicators that

- addressed an intervention with potential health benefits for the patient
- were supported by scientific evidence or formal professional consensus (guidelines, for example)
- can be significantly influenced by the health care delivery system
- can be assessed from available sources of information, primarily the medical record.

The literature review process varied slightly for each clinical area, but the basic strategy involved the following:

- Identify general areas in which quality indicators are likely to be developed.
- Review relevant textbooks and review articles.
- Conduct a targeted MEDLINE search on specific topics related to the probable indicator areas.

The levels of evidence for each indicator were assigned to three categories: randomized clinical trial; nonrandomized controlled trials, cohort or case analysis, or multiple time series; and textbooks, opinions, or descriptive studies. For each proposed indicator, staff noted the highest level of evidence supporting the indicator.

Because of the breadth of topics for which we were developing indicators, some of the literature reviews relied exclusively on textbooks and review articles. Nonetheless, we believe that the reviews adequately summarize clinical opinion and key research at the time that they were conducted. The literature reviews used to develop quality indicators for children and adolescents, and for women, were conducted between January and July 1995. The reviews for general medical conditions, oncologic conditions, and cardiopulmonary conditions were conducted between November 1996 and July 1997.

For each clinical area, we wrote a summary of the scientific evidence and developed tables of the proposed indicators that included the level of evidence, specific studies in support of the indicator, and the clinical rationale for the indicator. Because the organization of care delivery is changing so rapidly, we drafted indicators that were not in most cases inextricably linked to the place where the care was provided.

Types of Indicators

Quality of care is usually determined with three types of measures:

- *Structural measures* include characteristics of clinicians (for instance, board certification or years of experience), organizations (for instance, staffing patterns or types of equipment available), and patients (for instance, type of insurance or severity of illness).
- *Process measures* include the ways in which clinicians and patients interact and the appropriateness of medical treatment for a specific patient.
- *Outcomes measures* include changes in patients' current and future health status, including health-related quality of life and satisfaction with care.

The indicators included in the QA Tools system are primarily process indicators. We deliberately chose such indicators because the system was designed to assess care for which we can hold providers responsible. However, we collect data on a number of intermediate outcomes measures (for example, glycosylated hemoglobin, blood pressure, and cholesterol) that could be used to construct intermediate clinical outcomes indicators.

In many instances, the measures included in the QA Tools system are used to determine whether interventions have been provided in response to poor performance on such measures (for instance, whether persons who fail to control their blood sugar on dietary therapy are offered oral hypoglycemic therapy).

The Expert Panel Process

We convened expert panels to evaluate the indicators and to make final selections using the RAND/UCLA Appropriateness Method, a modified Delphi method developed at RAND and UCLA (Brook 1994). In general, the method quantitatively assesses the expert judgment of a group of clinicians regarding the indicators by using a scale with values ranging from 1 to 9.

The method is iterative with two rounds of anonymous ratings of the indicators by the panel and a face-to-face group discussion between rounds. Each panelist has equal weight in determining the final result: the quality indicators that will be included in the QA Tools system.

The RAND/UCLA Appropriateness Method has been shown to have a reproducibility consistent with that of well accepted diagnostic tests such as the interpretation of coronary angiography and screening mammography (Shekelle et al., 1998a). It has also been shown to have content, construct, and predictive validity in other applications (Brook, 1994; Shekelle et al., 1998b; Kravitz et al., 1995; Selby et al., 1996).

Approximately six weeks before the panel meeting, we sent panelists the reviews of the literature, the staff-proposed quality indicators, and separate rating sheets for each clinical area. We asked the panelists to examine the literature review and rate each indicator on a nine-point scale on each of two dimensions: validity and feasibility.

A quality indicator is defined as valid if:

1. Adequate scientific evidence or professional consensus exists supporting the indicator.

2. There are identifiable health benefits to patients who receive care specified by the indicator.

3. Based on the panelists' professional experience, health professionals with significantly higher rates of adherence to an indicator would be considered higher quality providers

4. The majority of factors that determine adherence to an indicator are under the control of the health professional (or are subject to influence by the health professional—for example, smoking cessation).

Ratings of 1-3 mean that the indicator is not a valid criterion for evaluating quality. Ratings of 4-6 mean that the indicator is an uncertain or equivocal criterion for evaluating quality. Ratings of 7-9 mean that the indicator is clearly a valid criterion for evaluating quality.

A quality indicator is defined as feasible if:

1. The information necessary to determine adherence is likely to be found in a typical medical record.

2. Estimates of adherence to the indicator based on medical record data are likely to be reliable and unbiased.

3. Failure to document relevant information about the indicator is itself a marker for poor quality.

Ratings of 1-3 mean that it is not feasible to use the indicator for evaluating quality. Ratings of 4-6 mean that there will be considerable variability in the feasibility of using the indicator to evaluate quality. Ratings of 7-9 mean that it is clearly feasible to use the indicator for evaluating quality.

The first round of indicators was rated by the panelists individually in their own offices. The indicators were returned to RAND staff and the results of the first round were summarized. We encouraged panelists to comment on the literature reviews, the definitions of key terms, and the indicators. We also encouraged them to suggest additions or deletions to the indicators.

At the panel meeting, participants discussed each clinical area in turn, focusing on the evidence, or lack thereof, that supports or refutes each indicator and the panelists' prior validity rankings. Panelists had before them the summary of the panel's first round ratings and a confidential reminder of their own ratings.

The summary consisted of a printout of the rating sheet with the distribution of ratings by panelists displayed above the rating line (without revealing the identity of the panelists) and a caret (^) marking the individual panelist's own rating in the first round displayed below the line. An example of the printout received by panelists is shown in Figure I.1.

```
Chapter 1
ASTHMA                             Validity          Feasibility
```

DIAGNOSIS

```
3. Spirometry should be measured in patients    1   1 2 3 1 1                    3 4 2
with chronic asthma at least every 2 years.   1 2 3 4 5 6 7 8 9    1 2 3 4 5 6 7 8 9  ( 1- 2)
                                                          ^                        ^
```

TREATMENT

```
7. Patients requiring chronic treatment with
systemic corticosteroids during any 12 month
period should have been prescribed inhaled
corticosteroids during the same 12 month              1 6   2                    2 3 4
period.                                       1 2 3 4 5 6 7 8 9    1 2 3 4 5 6 7 8 9  ( 3- 4)
                                                          ^                        ^
10. All patients seen for an acute asthma
exacerbation should be evaluated with a
complete history including all of the
following:                                        2 2 2   3          2 2   1 1 3
   a. time of onset                           1 2 3 4 5 6 7 8 9    1 2 3 4 5 6 7 8 9  ( 5- 6)
                                                          ^                        ^

                                                      4 1 4                    3 1 5
   b. all current medications                 1 2 3 4 5 6 7 8 9    1 2 3 4 5 6 7 8 9  ( 7- 8)
                                                          ^                        ^

   c. prior hospitalizations and emergency           5 1 3                    5 1 3
      department visits for asthma            1 2 3 4 5 6 7 8 9    1 2 3 4 5 6 7 8 9  ( 9-10)
                                                          ^                        ^

   d. prior episodes of respiratory              1 1 3 2 2          1   2   3 1 2
      insufficiency due to asthma             1 2 3 4 5 6 7 8 9    1 2 3 4 5 6 7 8 9  (11-12)
                                                          ^                        ^
```

```
Scales:  1 = low validity or feasibility; 9 = high validity or feasibility
```

Figure I.1 - Sample Panelist Summary Rating Sheet

Panelists were encouraged to bring to the discussion any relevant published information that the literature reviews had omitted. In a few cases, they supplied this information which was, in turn, discussed. In several cases, the indicators were reworded or otherwise clarified to better fit clinical judgment.

After further discussion, all indicators in each clinical area were re-ranked for validity. These final round rankings were analyzed in a manner similar to past applications of the RAND/UCLA Appropriateness Method (Park et al., 1986; Brook, 1994). The median panel rating and measure of dispersion were used to categorize indicators on validity.

We regarded panel members as being in *disagreement* when at least three members of the panel judged an indicator as being in the highest tertile of validity (that is, having a rating of 7, 8, or 9) and three members rated it as being in the lowest tertile of validity (1, 2, or 3) (Brook, 1994). Indicators with a median validity rating of 7 or higher without disagreement were included in the system.

We also obtained ratings from the panelists about the feasibility of obtaining the data necessary to score the indicators from medical. This was done to make explicit that failure to document key variables required to score an indicator would be treated as though the recommended care was not provided.

Although we do not intend for quality assessment to impose significant additional documentation burdens, we wanted the panel to acknowledge that documentation itself is an element of quality particularly when patients are treated by a team of health professionals. Because of the variability in documentation patterns and the opportunity to empirically evaluate feasibility, indicators with a median feasibility rating of 4 and higher were accepted into the system. Indicators had to satisfy both the validity and feasibility criteria.

Five expert panels were convened on the topics of children's care, care for women 18-50, general medicine for adults, oncologic conditions and HIV, and cardiopulmonary conditions.

The dates on which the panels were conducted are shown in Table I.2.

Table I.2

Dates Expert Panels Convened

Children	October 1995
Women	November 1995
Cardiopulmonary	September 1997
Oncology/HIV	October 1997
General Medicine	November 1997

Tables I.3 through I.6 summarize the distribution of indicators by level of evidence, type of care (preventive, acute, chronic), function of medicine (screening, diagnosis, treatment, follow-up, continuity), and modality (for example, history, physical examination, laboratory test, medication) (Malin et al., 2000; Schuster et al., 1997).

The categories were selected by the research team and reflect terminology commonly used by health services researchers to describe different aspects of health service delivery. The categories also reflect the areas in which we intend to develop aggregate quality of care scores. However, a significant benefit of the QA Tools system is its adaptability to other frameworks.

Note: In the following tables, the figures in some columns may not total exactly 100 percent due to the rounding of fractional numbers.

Table I.3
Distribution of Indicators (%) by Level of Evidence

Level of Evidence	Children	Women	Cancer/HIV	Cardio-pulmonary	General Medicine
Randomized trials	11	22	22	18	23
Nonrandomized trials	6	16	37	4	17
Descriptive studies	72	59	26	71	57
Added by panel	12	4	15	7	4
Total	101	101	100	100	101

Table I.4
Distribution of Indicators (%) by Type of Care

Type of Care	Children	Women	Cancer/HIV	Cardio-pulmonary	General Medicine
Preventive	30	11	20	3	18
Acute	36	49	7	26	38
Chronic	34	41	74	71	44
Total	100	101	101	100	100

Table I.5

Distribution of Indicators (%) by Function of Medicine

Function of Medicine	Children	Women	Cancer/HIV	Cardio-pulmonary	General Medicine
Screening	23	18	9	3	12
Diagnosis	31	30	27	54	41
Treatment	36	43	53	36	41
Follow-up	10	12	10	8	6
Total	100	103	99	101	100

Table I.6

Distribution of Indicators (%) by Modality

Modality	Children	Women	Cancer/HIV	Cardio-pulmonary	General Medicine
History	19	18	4	11	23
Physical	19	10	5	21	15
Lab/Radiology	21	23	24	23	18
Medication	25	29	25	25	26
Other	17	19	42	20	17
Total	101	99	100	100	99

DEVELOPING QUALITY INDICATORS FOR ONCOLOGIC CONDITIONS AND HIV

We now describe in more detail the process by which we developed quality indicators for oncologic conditions and HIV.

Selecting Clinical Areas

We began our selection of clinical areas by examining national data sources to identify the leading causes of mortality, morbidity, and functional limitation among adult men and women. The principal data sources for this review were Vital Statistics, the National Health Interview Survey (NHIS), the National Ambulatory Medical Care Survey (NAMCS), and the National Hospital Discharge Survey (NHDS).

From these data sources, we selected the conditions that represent the top causes of mortality, hospitalization, and outpatient visits. This process led to the selection of some areas that were developed for the women's care panel (McGlynn et al., 2000b).

To facilitate the review and rating process, we grouped the selected areas into three categories: cardiopulmonary conditions, oncologic conditions and HIV, and general medical conditions. Table I.7 lists the clinical areas covered by each of these categories. "Cancer Pain and Palliation" was not among the originally selected clinical areas, but was added during the panel process as a result of strong recommendations from several oncology panelists.

Table I.7

Clinical Areas Covered by Each Expert Panel

Cardiopulmonary (N=12)	Oncology and HIV (N=11)	General Medicine (N=22)
Asthma*	Breast Cancer Screening	Acne*
Atrial Fibrillation	Breast Cancer Diagnosis and Treatment*	Alcohol Dependence*
Cerebrovascular Disease	Cervical Cancer Screening*	Allergic Rhinitis*
Chronic Obstructive Pulmonary Disease	Colorectal Cancer Screening	Benign Prostatic Hyperplasia
Cigarette Counseling*	Colorectal Cancer Diagnosis and Treatment	Cataracts
Congestive Heart Failure	HIV Disease	Cholelithiasis
Coronary Artery Disease Diagnosis and Screening	Lung Cancer	Dementia
Coronary Artery Disease Prevention and Treatment	Prostate Cancer Screening	Depression*
Hyperlipidemia	Prostate Cancer Diagnosis and Treatment	Diabetes Mellitus*
Hypertension*	Skin Cancer Screening	Dyspepsia and Peptic Ulcer Disease
Pneumonia	Cancer Pain and Palliation	Hormone Replacement Therapy
Upper Respiratory Infections*		Headache*
		Hip Fracture
		Hysterectomy
		Inguinal Hernia
		Low Back Pain (Acute)*
		Orthopedic Conditions
		Osteoarthritis
		Preventive Care*
		Urinary Tract Infections*
		Vaginitis and Sexually Transmitted Diseases*
		Vertigo and Dizziness

* Previously addressed by the panel on quality of care for women (McGlynn et al., 2000b).

Conducting Literature Reviews

The literature reviews were conducted as described earlier in this Introduction by a team of 14 physician investigators, many of whom have clinical expertise in the conditions selected for this project. Each investigator drafted a review of the literature for his or her topic area, focusing on important areas for quality measurement (as opposed to a clinical review of the literature, which would focus on clinical management) and drafted potential indicators.

Every indicator table was then reviewed by Drs. Asch or Kerr for content, consistency, and the likely availability of information necessary to score adherence to the indicator from the medical record. On a few occasions, when questions remained even after detailed literature review, we requested that a clinical leader in the field read and comment on the draft review and indicators.

In addition, the physician investigators updated the 16 clinical areas carried over from the women's care panel. This included reading the reviews and indicators from the women's care panel, updating the supporting literature to 1997, and modifying the pre-existing indicators as appropriate. In most cases few changes were made, but indicators were deleted if the evidence changed or if our implementation experience proved that it was not feasible to collect the data necessary to determine eligibility and/or a scoring indicator. Indicators were added if strong evidence since 1995 supported the need for a new criterion. In the clinical areas previously addressed, the expert panels for this project rated only those indicators that had been added or significantly revised (indicated by bold type in the indicator tables in the chapters that follow).

This quality assessment system was designed to encompass a substantial portion of the inpatient and ambulatory care received by the population. In order to estimate the percentage of ambulatory care visits covered by this system, we aggregated applicable ICD-9 codes into the clinical areas for which we are developing quality indicators. We then calculated the number of adult visits for each condition in the 1993 National Ambulatory Medical Care Survey (NAMCS). We used the same method to estimate the percentage of inpatient admissions accounted for by each clinical area in the 1992 National Hospital Discharge Survey.

Aggregating ICD-9 codes into the clinical areas covered by this system was an imprecise task, requiring a rather broad definition of what is "included" in each clinical area. The 45 clinical conditions covered by this quality measurement system encompass 50 percent of all ambulatory care visits and 46 percent of non-federal inpatient hospital admissions.

Developing Indicators

In each clinical area, we developed indicators defining the explicit criteria by which quality of care would be evaluated. These indicators focus on technical processes of care for the various conditions and are organized by function: screening, diagnosis, treatment and follow-up. Although we have developed indicators across the continuum of management for each condition, we have not attempted to cover every important area or every possible clinical circumstance. The indicators were designed to apply to the average patient with the specified condition who is seeing the average physician.

Our approach makes a strong distinction between indicators of quality of care and practice guidelines (see Table I.8). While guidelines are intended to be comprehensive in scope, indicators are meant to apply to specific clinical circumstances in which there is believed to be a strong link between a measurable health care process and patient outcomes.

Indicators are not intended to measure all possible care for a condition. Furthermore, guidelines are intended to be applied prospectively at the individual patient level, whereas indicators are applied retrospectively and scored at an aggregate level. Finally, indicators must be written precisely in order to be *operationalized* (that is, to form useful measures of quality based on medical records or administrative data).

Table I.8

Clinical Guidelines versus Quality Indicators

Guidelines	Indicators
Comprehensive: Cover virtually all aspects of care for a condition.	**Targeted**: Apply to specific clinical circumstances in which there is evidence of a process-outcome link.
Prescriptive: Intended to influence provider behavior prospectively at the individual patient level.	**Observational**: Measure past provider behavior at an aggregate level.
Flexible: Intentionally allow room for clinical judgment and interpretation.	**Operational**: Precise language that can be applied systematically to medical records or administrative data.

The indicator tables at the end of each chapter of this book
- note the population to whom the indicators apply
- list the indicators themselves
- provide a "grade" for the strength of the evidence that supports each indicator

- list the specific literature used to support each indicator
- provide a statement of the health benefits of complying with each indicator
- include comments to further explain the purpose or reasoning behind each indicator.

Selecting Panel Participants

We requested nominations for potential expert panel participants from the relevant specialty societies for oncology and HIV: the American College of Physicians, American Academy of Family Physicians, American Geriatrics Society, American Cancer Society, American Society of Clinical Oncology, Infectious Disease Society of America, and the Society of General Internal Medicine. We received a total of 206 nominations for the panels on general internal medicine, oncology and HIV, and cardiopulmonary conditions.

Each nominee was sent a letter summarizing the purpose of the project and indicating which group recommended them. Interested candidates were asked to return a curriculum vitae and calendar with available dates. We received positive responses from 156 potential panelists. The quality of the recommended panelists was excellent.

We sought to ensure that each panel was diverse with respect to type of practice (academic, private practice, managed care organizational practice), geographic location, gender, and specialty. The oncology panel included seven oncologists and two general internists. Dr. Lodovicco Balducci, an oncologist, was selected by RAND staff to chair this panel (see the Acknowledgements earlier in this book for the list of panelists).

Selecting the Final Indicators

The panel process was conducted as described earlier in this Introduction.

During the course of the Oncology and HIV panel meeting, several panelists noted the rapidity with which clinical practice in this field is changing. Therefore, process of care criteria that represented standard practice at the time of the panel meeting may soon become obsolete as new practices are found to be efficacious.

For many patients, the best option may be enrollment in a clinical trial of a new therapy (where standard therapy is the randomized alternative). To ensure that the importance of clinical trials is recognized, we have included enrollment in such trials, with documentation of informed consent, as meeting the intent of several oncology indicators for which panelists felt this option was appropriate. For all other indicators included in the system, patients participating in a relevant clinical trial will be considered ineligible for the intervention specified in the indicator(s) and will not be included in the scoring.

Analyzing the Final Set of Indicators

A total of 145 quality indicators (including subparts) were reviewed by the oncology and HIV expert panel. All 11 indicators retained from the women's care panel were accepted by the oncology/HIV panel on the basis of the women's panel's ratings. Six indicators were deleted before the final panel ratings in response to revisions suggested by panelists prior to or during the panel meeting. Of the remaining 128 indicators that received final ratings from this panel, 20 were added by the oncology and HIV care panel itself. This occurred either when panelists agreed that a new indicator should be written to cover an important topic, or, more frequently, as a result of splitting a staff-proposed indicator.

The panel accepted 106 (83%) of the 128 indicators it rated. Twenty-two indicators (17%) were dropped due to low ratings: 17 for low validity scores, 3 for substantial disagreement on validity, and 2 for low feasibility scores.

Table I.9 summarizes the disposition of all 145 proposed oncology and HIV quality indicators by the strength of their supporting evidence. The final set consists of 117 indicators (106 rated by this panel and 11 approved based on ratings by the women's panel), or 81 percent of those proposed. Table I.9 reveals that indicators that are not based on randomized clinical trials (that is, Level II and Level III indicators) were much more likely to be rejected by the panel. Similarly, indicators proposed by the panelists themselves fared poorly relative to those with Level I evidence. This pattern has been observed consistently across several RAND quality of care panels.

Table I.9

**Disposition of Proposed Oncology and HIV Quality Indicators
by Strength of Evidence**

Strength of Evidence	Total Proposed	Indicator Disposition			
		Accepted	Retained from Women's Panel	Drop before Rating	Drop Due to Low Rating
I. Randomized controlled trials	27 (100%)	26 (96%)	0 (0%)	0 (0%)	1 (4%)
II. Non-randomized trials	57 (100%)	41 (72%)	2 (4%)	2 (4%)	12 (21%)
III. Opinions, descriptive studies, or textbooks	41 (100%)	22 (54%)	9 (22%)	4 (10%)	6 (15%)
IV. Added by Clinical Panel	20 (100%)	17 (85%)	0 (0%)	0 (0%)	3 (15%)
Total	**145 (100%)**	**106 (73%)**	**11 (8%)**	**6 (4%)**	**22 (15%)**

The summary ratings sheets for oncology and HIV are shown in Appendix A of this book.

Figure I.2 provides an example of a final summary rating sheet. The chapter number and clinical condition are shown in the top left margin. The rating bar is numbered from 1 to 9, indicating the range of possible responses. The number shown above each of the responses in the rating bar indicates how many panelists provided that particular rating for the indicator. Below the score distribution, in parentheses, the median and the absolute deviation from the media are listed. Each dimension is assigned an A for "Agreement", D for "Disagreement", or I for "Indeterminate" based on the score distribution.

Note: We recommend caution when reviewing the ratings for each indicator. The overall median does not tell us anything about the extent to which the indicators occur in clinical practice. To determine that, actual clinical data to assess the indicators must be collected and analyzed.

1. HIV+ patients should be offered PCP prophylaxis within one month of meeting any of the following conditions:

```
                                              1 8              3 6
a. CD4 count dropping below 200     1 2 3 4 5 6 7 8 9   1 2 3 4 5 6 7 8 9   ( 1- 2)
                                      (9.0, 0.1, A)       (9.0, 0.3, A)
                                    2 1 2  1 1    2     2        1 1 1 2 2
b. Thrush                           1 2 3 4 5 6 7 8 9   1 2 3 4 5 6 7 8 9   ( 3- 4)
                                      (3.0, 2.2, I)       (7.0, 2.3, I)
                                                2 7              3 6
c. Completion of active treatment   1 2 3 4 5 6 7 8 9   1 2 3 4 5 6 7 8 9   ( 5- 6)
   of PCP                             (9.0, 0.2, A)       (9.0, 0.3, A)
                                            1 1 1 6          3 6
d.  CD4 below 15%                    1 2 3 4 5 6 7 8 9   1 2 3 4 5 6 7 8 9   ( 7- 8)
                                      (9.0, 0.7, A)       (9.0, 0.3, A)
```

2. HIV+ patients who do not have active TB and who have not ever previously received TB prophylaxis should be offered TB prophylaxis within one month of meeting any of following conditions:

```
                                              1 3 5            1 3 5
a. Current PPD > 5 mm               1 2 3 4 5 6 7 8 9   1 2 3 4 5 6 7 8 9   ( 9-10)
                                      (9.0, 0.6, A)       (9.0, 0.6, A)
b. Provider noting that patient
   has had PPD                            2 4 3         1   1 3 1 3
> 5 mm administered at anytime      1 2 3 4 5 6 7 8 9   1 2 3 4 5 6 7 8 9   (11-12)
   since HIV diagnosis                (8.0, 0.6, A)       (7.0, 1.2, A)
                                    2  1 1  1 2 2     2   1 2 1 3
c. Contact with person with         1 2 3 4 5 6 7 8 9   1 2 3 4 5 6 7 8 9   (13-14)
   active TB                          (7.0, 2.7, D)       (4.0, 1.6, I)
```

3. HIV+ patients who do not have active toxoplasmosis should be offered toxoplasmosis prophylaxis within one month of meeting either of the following conditions:

```
- Toxo IgG positive and CD4 count dropping
  below 100
- Completion of therapy for active        3   6              2 2 5
  toxoplasmosis                    1 2 3 4 5 6 7 8 9   1 2 3 4 5 6 7 8 9   (15-16)
                                      (9.0, 0.7, A)       (9.0, 0.7, A)
```

4. HIV+ patients should have toxoplasmosis serology documented.

```
                                            4 1 4            3 4 2
                                    1 2 3 4 5 6 7 8 9   1 2 3 4 5 6 7 8 9   (17-18)
                                      (8.0, 0.9, A)       (8.0, 0.6, A)
```

5. HIV+ patients should be offered MAC prophylaxis within one month of a CD4 count dropping below 50.

```
                                            2 2 5            3 2 4
                                    1 2 3 4 5 6 7 8 9   1 2 3 4 5 6 7 8 9   (19-20)
                                      (9.0, 0.7, A)       (8.0, 0.8, A)
```

6. HIV+ patients with a lowest recorded CD4 > 200 should have a documented pneumovax.

```
                                          1 3 3 2       1      1 5   2
                                    1 2 3 4 5 6 7 8 9   1 2 3 4 5 6 7 8 9   (21-22)
                                      (8.0, 0.8, A)       (7.0, 1.1, A)
```

7. HIV+ patients with a lowest recorded CD4 count of less than 100 should have had a yearly dilated fundoscopic exam.

```
                                            4 2 3          1 2 3 3
                                    1 2 3 4 5 6 7 8 9   1 2 3 4 5 6 7 8 9   (23-24)
                                      (8.0, 0.8, A)       (8.0, 0.8, A)
```

8. HIV+ patients should have a VDRL or RPR documented in the chart.

```
                                          3 2 4            2 3 4
                                    1 2 3 4 5 6 7 8 9   1 2 3 4 5 6 7 8 9   (25-26)
                                      (8.0, 0.8, A)       (8.0, 0.7, A)
```

9. Sexually active HIV+ patients should be offered a VDRL/RPR annually.

```
                                    7    1    1       5 1 1    2
                                    1 2 3 4 5 6 7 8 9   1 2 3 4 5 6 7 8 9   (27-28)
                                      (1.0, 1.0, A)       (1.0, 1.2, A)
```

Scales: 1 = low validity or feasibility; 9 = high validity or feasibility

Figure I.2 - Sample Rating Results Sheet

The tables in Appendix B show the changes made to each indicator during the panel process, the reasons for those changes, and the final disposition of each indicator. Wherever possible, we have tried to briefly summarize the discussion that led the panel to either modify or drop indicators. These explanations are based on extensive notes taken by RAND staff during the panel process, but should not be considered representative of the views of all of the panelists, nor of any individual.

Because the final quality assessment system will produce aggregate scores for various dimensions of health care, it is useful to examine the distribution of the final indicators across some of these dimensions. Table I.10 summarizes the distribution of quality indicators by type of care (preventive, acute, and chronic), the function of the medical care provided (screening, diagnosis, treatment, and follow-up), and the modality by which care is delivered (history, physical examination, laboratory or radiologic study, medication, other interventions,[1] and other contacts[2]). Indicators were assigned to only one type of care, but could have up to two functions and three modalities.

Indicators with more than one function or modality were allocated fractionally across categories. For example, one indicator states, "For patients who present with a complaint of sore throat, a history/physical exam should document presence or absence of: a) fever; b) tonsillar exudate; c) anterior cervical adenopathy." This indicator was allocated 50 percent to the history modality and 50 percent to the physical examination modality.

---

[1] Other interventions include counseling, education, procedures, and surgery.
[2] Other contacts include general follow-up visit or phone call, referral to subspecialist, or hospitalization.

Table I.10

**Distribution of Final Oncology and HIV Quality
Indicators by Type of Care, Function, and Modality**

	Number of Indicators	Percent of Indicators
Type		
Preventive	23	20%
Acute	8	7%
Chronic	86	74%
Function		
Screening	11	9%
Diagnosis	32	27%
Treatment	62	53%
Follow-up	12	10%
Modality*		
History	5	4%
Physical Examination	6	5%
Laboratory or Radiologic Study	28	24%
Medication	29	25%
Other Intervention	50	43%
Other Contact	0	0%
Total	**117**	**100%**

* Total does not sum to 117 due to rounding.

CONCLUSION

This report provides the foundation for a broad set of quality indicators covering oncology and HIV health care. The final indicators presented here cover a variety of clinical conditions, span a range of clinical functions and modalities, and are rated by the level of evidence in the supporting literature. When combined with the indicators approved by the women's care, child and adolescent care, cardiopulmonary, and general medicine expert panels, the complete quality assessment system will be more comprehensive than any quality assessment system in use today.

The comprehensive nature of this system is demonstrated by the broad scope of the indicators. Of the 145 indicators reviewed by the oncology and HIV expert panel, 117 (81%) were retained. These indicators cover a mix of preventive, acute, and chronic care. However, given the chronic nature of the

conditions covered by this panel, a large proportion of the indicators (74%)
fall into the chronic care category. They address all four functions of
medicine, including screening, diagnosis, treatment and follow-up. Moreover,
the indicators cover a variety of modes of care provision, such as history,
physical examination, laboratory study, and medication. Many of the
oncology/HIV indicators (42%) are in the "Other Intervention" modality, which
includes surgery and radiation therapy.

There are many advantages to a comprehensive quality assessment system.
Not only does it cover a broad range of health conditions experienced by the
population, but it is also designed to detect underutilization of needed
services. In addition, because of its broad scope, it will be difficult for
health care organizations to improve their quality scores by focusing their
improvement efforts on only a few indicators or clinical areas.

Finally, this system can be effective for both internal and external
quality reviews. Sufficient clinical detail exists in the system such that
organizations will be able to use the resulting information to improve care,
while the simple summary scores that the system generates will be an important
tool for health care purchasers and consumers.

ORGANIZATION OF THIS DOCUMENT

The rest of this volume is organized as follows:

- Each chapter summarizes:
  - Results of the literature review for one condition.
  - Provides a table of the staff's recommended indicators based on
    that review.
  - Indicates the level of scientific evidence supporting each
    indicator along with the specific relevant citations.
- *Appendix A* provides the summary rating sheets for each condition.
- *Appendix B* shows the changes made to each indicator during the panel
  process, the reasons for those changes, and the final disposition of
  each indicator.

REFERENCES

Brook, R. H., "The RAND/UCLA Appropriateness Method," *Clinical Practice Guideline Development: Methodology Perspectives*, AHCPR Pub. No. 95-0009, Rockville, MD: Public Health Service, 1994.

Kerr E. A., S. M. Asch, E. G. Hamilton, E. A. McGlynn (eds.), *Quality of Care for Cardiopulmonary Conditions: A Review of the Literature and Quality Indicators*, Santa Monica, CA: RAND, MR-1282-AHRQ, 2000a.

Kerr E. A., S. M. Asch, E. G. Hamilton, E. A. McGlynn (eds.), *Quality of Care for General Medical Conditions: A Review of the Literature and Quality Indicators*, Santa Monica, CA: RAND, MR-1280-AHRQ, 2000b.

Kravitz R. L., M. Laouri, J. P. Kahan, P. Guzy, et al., "Validity of Criteria Used for Detecting Underuse of Coronary Revascularization," *JAMA* 274(8):632-638, 1995.

Malin, J. L., S. M. Asch, E. A. Kerr, E. A. McGlynn. "Evaluating the Quality of Cancer Care: Development of Cancer Quality Indicators for a Global Quality Assessment Tool," *Cancer* 88:701-7, 2000.

McGlynn E. A., C. Damberg, E. A. Kerr, M. Schuster (eds.), *Quality of Care for Children and Adolescents: A Review of Selected Clinical Conditions and Quality Indicators*, Santa Monica, CA: RAND, MR-1283-HCFA, 2000a.

McGlynn E. A., E. A. Kerr, C. Damberg, S. M. Asch (eds.), *Quality of Care for Women: A Review of Selected Clinical Conditions and Quality Indicators*, Santa Monica, CA: RAND, MR-1284-HCFA, 2000b.

Park R. A., Fink A., Brook R. H., Chassin M. R., et al., "Physician Ratings of Appropriate Indications for Six Medical and Surgical Procedures," *AJPH* 76(7):766-772, 1986.

Schuster M. A., S. M. Asch, E. A. McGlynn, et al., "Development of a Quality of Care Measurement System for Children and Adolescents: Methodological

Considerations and Comparisons With a System for Adult Women," *Archives of Pediatrics and Adolescent Medicine* 151:1085-1092, 1997.

Selby J. V., B. H. Fireman, R. J. Lundstrom, et al., "Variation among Hospitals in Coronary-Angiography Practices and Outcomes after Myocardial Infarction in a Large Health Maintenance Organization," *N Engl J Med* 335:1888-96, 1996.

Shekelle P. G., J. P. Kahan, S. J. Bernstein, et al., "The Reproducibility of a Method to Identify the Overuse and Underuse of Medical Procedures," *N Engl J Med,* 338:1888-1895, 1998b.

Shekelle P. G., M. R. Chassin, R. E. Park, "Assessing the Predictive Validity of the RAND/UCLA Appropriateness Method Criteria for Performing Carotid Endarterectomy," *Int J Technol Assess Health Care* 14(4):

1. BREAST CANCER SCREENING

Deidre Gifford, MD, MPH

The literature for this chapter was identified by a MEDLINE search for English language review articles on breast cancer screening from 1992 to the present, and by reviewing the U.S. Preventive Services Task Force Guide to Clinical Preventive Services (USPSTF, 1996). Once general topics for indicators were selected, additional articles reporting primary data on the topics were identified based on the bibliographies of the review articles and the USPSTF chapter and reviewed. In addition, a focused search for randomized trials of breast self-examination (BSE) was performed.

IMPORTANCE

Breast cancer is the most commonly diagnosed nondermatologic cancer and the second leading cause of cancer-related deaths among women in the United States (MMWR, 1996). In 1995, there were an estimated 182,000 newly diagnosed cases and 46,000 deaths from breast cancer in the U.S. (USPSTF, 1996). An estimated 12 percent of all U.S. women will be given the diagnosis during their lifetime, and 3.5 percent will die of this disease (Harris et al., 1992). Furthermore, the incidence of breast cancer is rising, with an increase of 55 percent between 1950 and 1991. For women, breast cancer is surpassed only by motor vehicle injury and infection as a cause for potential years of life lost before age 65 (USPSTF, 1996).

SCREENING

There are three principle methods available for breast cancer screening. These include periodic BSE, clinical breast examination (CBE), and screening mammography. The goal of all three methods is to detect breast cancer at an earlier stage than it would have been detected had the screening method not been used. Earlier detection of breast cancers is hypothesized to lead to higher detection of cancers before systemic involvement has occurred, leading to decreased mortality (Harris et al., 1992).

There are limited data on the effectiveness of BSE in reducing mortality from breast cancer. One prospective non-randomized trial in the United

Kingdom compared breast cancer mortality in communities that received a BSE educational intervention with communities that did not (Ellman et al., 1993). There was no reduction in breast cancer mortality in the BSE communities at ten years of follow-up. The relative risk (RR) of death from breast cancer in the BSE groups was 1.01, with a 95 percent confidence interval (CI) of 0.86 to 1.17. Some retrospective studies have suggested that women who practice BSE present with earlier stage disease and less systemic involvement than those who do not, but other studies have found no effect (Baines, 1994). The additional benefit of BSE in populations already being screened with combinations of CBE and mammography is also not clear. The American Academy of Family Practice, American College of Obstetricians and Gynecologists (ACOG) and the American Cancer Society currently recommend teaching patients BSE, whereas the 1996 USPSTF report states that the evidence supporting the routine teaching of BSE is insufficient.

Data about the effectiveness of CBE alone or in combination with mammography are inconclusive. Seven randomized trials have compared the effectiveness of mammography with or without CBE to no screening; no studies have directly compared annual CBE to no screening. The Health Insurance Plan of Greater New York trial compared annual mammography plus annual CBE with no screening in women aged 40 to 64 years at study entry (Shapiro et al., 1988). At 18 years of follow-up, there was a 20 percent reduction in breast cancer mortality in the screened group. Although the incremental benefit of CBE cannot be directly determined from this trial, modeling studies have suggested that two-thirds of the effectiveness may have been due to CBE (Eddy, 1989). In contrast to these findings of potential benefit to CBE, a meta-analysis of the seven mammography/CBE trials in women aged 40 to 79 reported similar reductions in breast cancer mortality between those screened with mammography alone (RR 0.78) and those screened with mammography plus CBE (RR 0.79) (Kerlikowske et al., 1995). The American Cancer Society, American College of Radiology, American Medical Association, and ACOG recommend annual CBE beginning at age 40. The USPSTF states that there is insufficient evidence to recommend for or against routine CBE in women aged 40 to 49, or on the use of screening CBE alone (without mammography).

The effectiveness of screening mammography in women between the ages of 50 and 69 in reducing mortality from breast cancer has been documented by

several randomized trials (Kerlikowske et al., 1995; USPSTF, 1996).
Mammography with or without CBE reduces mortality from breast cancer by 20 to
30 percent in this age group. The optimal screening interval has not been
established. Although annual screening is recommended by many groups (USPSTF,
1996), the meta-analysis of seven randomized trials found equivalent mortality
reductions in women screened every 12 months (RR 0.77) and women screened
every 18 to 33 months (RR 0.77) (Kerlikowske et al., 1995). The USPSTF
recommends routine screening with mammography alone or mammography and annual
CBE in women aged 50 to 69 (Indicator 1).

The effectiveness of routine mammography screening in women over age 69
has not been clearly established in randomized trials. None of the seven
randomized clinical trials included women over age 74 at study entry. The
Swedish two-county trial included women aged 70 to 74 and found no difference
in the risk of breast cancer mortality between the group screened with
mammography alone every 24 to 33 months and those not screened at all (RR
0.98; 95% CI 0.63-1.53, the wide confidence interval reflects the small number
of women in this sub-group analysis) (Tabar, 1992). Among all subjects aged
40 to 74 at study entry, the two-county trial did show a significant reduction
in breast cancer mortality. Breast cancer is prevalent in women over age 65,
with 40 percent of cases occurring in this age group (Satariano, 1992). There
is no evidence that mammography is less sensitive in this population, as there
is in women under age 50 (USPSTF, 1996); however, with increasing age the
added benefit of early diagnosis of breast cancer may be offset by competing
morbidities, such that screening may be more beneficial in healthier older
women than in those with many co-morbid conditions (Mor, 1992). The USPSTF
guidelines state that although randomized trials have not yet shown a clear
benefit of screening in this population, "recommendations for screening women
aged 70 and over who have a reasonable life expectancy may be made based on
other grounds, such as the high burden of suffering in this age group and the
lack of evidence of differences in mammogram test characteristics in older
women versus those age 50-69." Organizations such as the American Cancer
Society, American College of Radiology, American Medical Association, and ACOG
do not specify an upper age limit for screening in their recommendations.

Sub-group analyses of those randomized trials including women aged 40 to
49 at study entry do not clearly show a reduction in mortality in this age

group (RR 0.93; 95% CI 0.76-1.13). In the subgroup of women aged 40 to 49 at study entry who had two-view mammography and 10 to 12 years of follow-up, the mortality RR was 0.73 (95% CI 0.54-1.00) (Kerlikowske et al., 1995). This marginally significant finding suggests that the benefits of screening in women aged 40 to 49 may not be realized until longer follow-up times have been achieved; however, it is possible that the same result could be obtained if screening began at age 50. The USPSTF considers the evidence insufficient to recommend periodic mammography in women aged 40 to 49.

REFERENCES

Baines CJ. 1994. The Canadian National Breast Screening Study: A Perspective on Criticisms. *Archives of Internal Medicine* 120: 326-34.

Breast Cancer Incidence and Mortality - United States 1992. 1996. *Morbidity and Mortality Weekly Report* 45 (39): 833-51.

Eddy DM. 1989. Screening for Breast Cancer. *Archives of Internal Medicine* 111: 389-99.

Ellman R, Moss SM, Coleman D, and Chamberlain J. 1993. Breast self-examination programmes in the trial of early detection of breast cancer: ten-year findings. *British Journal of Cancer* 68: 208-12.

Harris JR, Lippman ME, Veronesi U, and Willett W. 1992. Breast Cancer. *New England Journal of Medicine* 327 (5): 319-26.

Kerlikowske K, Grady D, Rubin S, et al. 1995. Efficacy of Screening Mammography: A Meta-analysis. *Journal of the American Medical Association* 273 (2): 149-53.

Mor V, Pacala JT, and Rakowski W. 1992. Mammography for Older Women: Who Uses, Who Benefits? *Journal of Gerontology* 47: 43-49.

Satariano WA. 1992. Comorbidity and Functional Status in Older Women With Breast Cancer: Implications for Screening, Treatment, and Prognosis. *Journal of Gerontology* 47: 24-31.

Shapiro S, Venet W, Strax P, et al. 1988. *Periodic screening for breast cancer*. Baltimore: Johns Hopkins University Press.

Tabar L, Fagerberg G, Duffy S, et al. 1992. Update of the Swedish Two-County Program of Mammographic Screening For Breast Cancer. *Radiologic Clinics of North America* 30 (1): 187-92.

US Preventative Services Task Force. 1996. *Guide to Clinical Preventative Services, 2nd ed*. Baltimore: Williams & Wilkins.

QUALITY INDICATORS FOR BREAST CANCER SCREENING

The following indicators apply to women age 18 and over.

Indicator	Quality of Evidence	Literature	Benefits	Comments
1. Women age 52 to 69 should have had a screening mammography performed in the past 2 years.	I	Kerlikowske et al., 1995; USPSTF, 1996.	Reduce breast cancer mortality.	Meta-analysis of seven randomized trials shows that periodic screening mammography in this age group, with or without CBE , leads to a reduction in breast cancer mortality of 20-30%. Starting at age 52 ensures that the women eligible for this indicator have been over age 50 for at least 2 years.

Quality of Evidence Codes

I	RCT
II-1	Nonrandomized controlled trials
II-2	Cohort or case analysis
II-3	Multiple time series
III	Opinions or descriptive studies

2.   BREAST CANCER DIAGNOSIS AND TREATMENT[1]

Deidre Gifford MD, MPH and Lisa Schmidt, MPH

The literature for this chapter was identified by a MEDLINE search of English language review articles from 1992 to the present on the subjects of breast mass, breast cancer treatment, and breast cancer follow-up. Consensus statements and guidelines on the subject were also reviewed, after which topics for indicators were developed. Randomized trials and meta-analyses pertinent to the indicators were then examined to verify the information contained in the reviews and to finalize the indicators. The topic of screening for breast cancer is covered in Chapter 1.

IMPORTANCE

See Chapter 1 for a discussion of the importance of breast cancer.

DIAGNOSIS

Clinical examination of the breast can detect a mass, but it is not sufficient to distinguish a benign from a malignant process (Donegan, 1992). Although characteristics such as indistinct borders, skin dimpling, or nipple retraction may distinguish breast cancer from a benign mass, the absence of these characteristics cannot reliably differentiate a benign mass from a malignant tumor. In addition, a clinical exam cannot distinguish a cystic from a solid breast mass (Donegan, 1992).

The American College of Obstetricians and Gynecologists (ACOG) recommends that all positive findings from a breast examination be documented in writing or with an appropriate drawing in the patient's chart (ACOG, 1991). In addition, a comprehensive history, including age, menstrual status, parity, previous history of breast-feeding, family medical history, and drug usage should be noted (Bland and Love, 1992).

Some type of follow-up should be provided for all women with a breast mass detected by physical examination (Indicator 1). Bland and Love (1992)

---

[1] This chapter is a revision of one written for an earlier project on quality of care for women and children (Q1). The expert panel for the current project was asked to review all of the indicators, but only rated new or revised indicators.

and Dixon and Mansel (1994) recommend fine needle aspiration (FNA) for any palpable breast mass (Indicator 2). Cytologic examination and FNA have been shown to be efficacious, cost-effective, and highly reliable when cytologic preparation and cellular sampling are properly done (Bland and Love, 1992) (Indicator 3). Aspiration is also effective for differentiating a cyst from a solid mass (Donegan, 1992). If the FNA cannot rule out breast cancer, an open biopsy should be performed (ACOG, 1994) (Indicator 4). In addition, ACOG (1991) suggests that any of the following findings on FNA requires that an open biopsy be performed:

- Bloody cyst fluid on aspiration;
- Failure of mass to disappear completely upon fluid aspiration;
- Recurrence of cyst after one or two aspirations;
- Solid dominant mass not diagnosed as fibroadenoma;
- Bloody nipple discharge;
- Nipple ulceration or persistent crusting; or
- Skin edema and erythema suggestive of inflammatory breast carcinoma.

Mammography is an essential part of the examination of a palpable breast mass (ACOG, 1994; Donegan, 1992). Significant mammographic findings are alterations in breast tissue density, calcifications, skin thickening, fibrous streaks, and nipple discharge (ACOG, 1991). However, mammography alone is not sufficient to rule out malignant pathology. Ultrasonography or magnified mammographic imaging of the breast may provide additional information and identify cysts or variations in normal breast architecture that account for the palpable abnormality (ACOG, 1994). Sonograms cannot distinguish benign from malignant masses, although they can accurately identify masses as cystic or solid (Donegan, 1992) (Indicator 3b). Sonograms are most helpful when a mass cannot be felt, when the patient will not permit aspiration, or when a mass is too small and deep to offer a reliable target for aspiration (Donegan, 1992).

The combination of physical examination, mammography, and FNA is highly accurate when all the tests give the same results (Donegan, 1992). A study discussed by Donegan (1992) found cancer in only three of 457 cases in which all three evaluations indicated that a mass was benign.

TREATMENT

The principal treatment for breast cancer in this century has been radical mastectomy. Breast cancer was believed to be a local/regional disease process that was best treated by aggressive local excision. More recently, treatment has moved toward a more conservative surgical approach, with adjuvant systemic therapy for women with evidence of spread of the disease to regional lymph nodes (Hortobagyi and Buzdar, 1995; National Institutes of Health, 1990).

Clinical staging of breast cancer uses the Tumor, Nodes, Metastases (TNM) system. This process assesses the tumor size, level of lymph node involvement, and presence or absence of metastases. Tables 2.1 and 2.2 show the definitions used for breast cancer staging.

Table 2.1

Definitions for Breast Cancer Staging

Tumor

TIS	Carcinoma in situ (intraductal carcinoma, lobular)
T0	No evidence of primary tumor
T1	Tumor $\leq$ 2cm in greatest dimension
T2	Tumor > 2cm but $\leq$ 5cm in greatest dimension
T3	Tumor > 5cm in greatest dimension
T4	Tumor of any size with direct extension into chest wall or skin

Nodes

N0	No regional lymph node metastases
N1	Metastases to movable ipsilateral axillary node(s)
N2	Metastases to ipsilateral axillary lymph node(s), fixed to one another or other structures
N3	Metastases to ipsilateral internal mammary lymph nodes

Metastases

M0	No distant metastases
M1	Distant metastases including ipsilateral supraclavicular nodes

Source: Adapted from Philips and Balducci (1996)

Table 2.2

Classification of Breast Cancer Stages

Stage 0:	TIS N0 M0
Stage I:	T1 N0 M0
Stage IIA:	T0 N1 M0, T1 N1 M0, T2 N0 M0
Stage IIB:	T2 N1 M0, T3 N0 M0
Stage IIIA:	T0 N2 M0, T1 N2 M0, T2 N2 M0, T3 N1/2 M0
Stage IIIB:	T4, any N, M0; *or* any T, N3
Stage IV:	Any T, any N, M1

Source: Adapted from Philips and Balducci (1996)

Surgical Treatment

In 1990, a National Institutes of Health (NIH) consensus panel reviewed the surgical treatment of early stage breast cancer (Stages I and II). In 1992, a consensus statement by four professional societies -- the American College of Radiology, American College of Surgeons, College of American Pathologists and Society of Surgical Oncology -- reviewed the literature and concurred with the NIH consensus (Winchester, 1992). Both of these consensus panels reviewed the results of seven randomized controlled trials with up to 17 years of follow-up comparing mastectomy with breast-conservation treatment in conjunction with whole breast irradiation. Breast conservation is defined as the excision of the primary breast tumor and adjacent breast tissue (breast-conserving surgery) and the dissection of ipsilateral lymph nodes, followed by irradiation. Breast-conserving surgery is also commonly referred to as lumpectomy, partial mastectomy, and segmental mastectomy (Winchester, 1992). Modified radical mastectomy involves removal of the entire breast with dissection of ipsilateral lymph nodes. All seven trials found that relapse-free survival and overall survival for both breast conservation and mastectomy were the same. From these results, the NIH consensus and the professional society consensus concluded that primary treatment for Stage I or II breast cancer can include *either* modified radical mastectomy *or* breast conservation treatment (Indicator 5). According to the NIH, no subgroups have been identified in which radiation therapy can be avoided after breast-conserving surgery (Indicators 6 and 7).

According to the NIH consensus, important considerations in the choice of surgical therapy for women with Stage I or II breast cancer include factors that influence local/regional tumor control, cosmetic results, psychosocial issues, and patient preferences for treatment method. Women with multicentric breast malignancies, including those with gross multifocal disease or diffuse microcalcifications detected by mammography, were believed to be inappropriate candidates for breast-conserving treatment, as were women for whom "breast conservation treatment would produce an unacceptable cosmetic result (e.g., women with large tumors relative to breast size and those with certain collagen vascular diseases)." In all other cases, the NIH suggests that "women should be educated about treatment choices and clinical trial options in order to make an informed decision in consultation with their physicians. A woman's body image and her beliefs and concerns may determine her preference for breast conservation treatment or mastectomy." In keeping with this recommendation of the NIH, the professional society consensus states that an assessment of the patient's needs and expectations is critical in patient selection for breast conservation treatment, as are a history and physical exam, mammography, and histologic assessment of the resected breast specimen (Winchester, 1992).

Adjuvant Systemic Therapy

In the 1970s, randomized clinical trials began to examine the benefits of adjuvant systemic therapy for women with early stage breast cancer. Early trials demonstrated that 1) adjuvant chemotherapy improved disease-free and overall survival; 2) adjuvant tamoxifen improved disease-free and overall survival; and 3) ovarian ablation prolonged disease-free and, sometimes, overall survival for premenopausal women (Hortobagyi and Buzdar, 1995). In 1985, and again in 1990, the Early Breast Cancer Trialists Collaborative Group (EBCTCG) performed a meta-analysis of all available randomized trials of adjuvant systemic therapy in early stage breast cancer begun before 1985. They pooled the results of 133 studies involving 75,000 women, which provided greater statistical power than individual studies to examine results (EBCTCG, 1992). This meta-analysis established that adjuvant chemotherapy or adjuvant tamoxifen produced significant reductions in the annual odds of recurrence and the annual odds of death compared with no adjuvant systemic treatment. It also confirmed that combination chemotherapy was superior to single-agent chemotherapy (EBCTCG, 1992; Hortobagyi and Buzdar, 1995).

Tamoxifen

Results of the EBCTCG meta-analysis showed reductions of 25 percent in the annual odds of recurrence and 17 percent in the annual odds of death for all women treated with tamoxifen. Both of these findings were statistically significant (p<0.00001). Ten year recurrence-free survival was 51 percent in the tamoxifen groups and 44 percent in controls (p<0.00001). Overall survival at ten years was 59 percent in the tamoxifen groups and 53 percent in the controls (p<0.00001). When the results were stratified by age, the analysis showed that the reduction in the odds of death occurred only for women over 50 years old, while the reduction in recurrence was seen in all age groups. This result, however, should be interpreted with caution, because the number of women in the tamoxifen trials below the age of 50 was smaller than the number of women over age 50 (8,612 vs. 21,280). The proportional risk reductions for both overall survival and recurrence-free survival were the same in node-negative and node-positive women, but because recurrence is generally more common in node-positive women, the absolute reduction in recurrence and death is greater in the node-positive group (Indicator 7). The EBCTG found a greater increase in recurrence-free survival in those trials which used >= two years of Tamoxifen compared to those which used less than two years (Indicator

7). Randomized trials are currently underway to study the optimal duration of Tamoxifen therapy (Current Trials Working Party of the Cancer Research Campaign Breast Cancer Trials Group, 1996).

Combination Chemotherapy

The EBCTCG overview reported the results of 31 randomized trials that included 11,000 women undergoing long-term (greater than two months) combination chemotherapy versus no chemotherapy. The median duration of treatment in these trials was 12 months. Five year recurrence-free survival was 59 percent in the chemotherapy groups versus 50 percent in the no chemotherapy group, a statistically significant reduction in recurrence of nine percent at five years. This difference persisted, but did not increase at ten year follow-up. Ten year overall survival in the chemotherapy group was 51 percent vs. 45 percent in the no chemotherapy group, again a statistically significant reduction in deaths for the chemotherapy group. When stratified by nodal status, the recurrence-free survival was increased by nearly nine percent in node-positive women, and by seven percent in node-negative women. Overall survival at ten years was better by seven percent for node-positive women, and by four percent for node-negative women. All improvements in outcome for both node-positive and node-negative women were statistically significant (Indicator 7).

Ovarian Ablation

Results are available for 12 trials involving 3,000 women comparing ovarian ablation with no ablation. After 15 years, 53 percent of ovarian ablation patients and 42 percent of controls were alive and free of recurrence, for a statistically significant difference between groups of 11 percent. Among the 1,326 women over the age of 50, there was no significant effect of ovarian ablation on recurrence-free survival or overall survival. The effects in women under the age of 50 were highly statistically significant. For these women, as seen in the other analyses, the magnitude of the absolute benefit is likely to depend on nodal status. Among node-positive women less than 50 years old, the increases in recurrence-free survival (11%) and overall survival (13%) were significant. For node-negative women less than 50 years old, the number that died or had a recurrence was smaller, so the effects of treatment are not as reliably known.

Summary of Adjuvant Treatment

Both tamoxifen and combination chemotherapy have been shown to produce statistically significant increases in survival in all women with breast cancer. Ovarian ablation produces statistically significant reductions in recurrence and mortality in women under the age of 50.

The absolute reductions in recurrence and mortality are greatest in women with node-positive disease, since the absolute risk of recurrence or death is greatest in this group. However, some reduction in recurrence and death can also be expected in women with node-negative disease. In these women, since the absolute risk of recurrence is small, the risk/benefit ratio of adjuvant systemic treatment needs to be considered (NIH Consensus, 1990). Among women with node negative disease, characteristics such as overall health and menopausal status, and indicators of prognosis such as tumor size and nuclear grade may be used to inform the choice of adjuvant therapy.

FOLLOW-UP

In the past, intensive follow-up of women after primary treatment for breast cancer was recommended. Such follow-up often included the use of bone scans, chest x-rays, liver sonograms and other imaging, and was felt to lead to earlier detection of recurrence and improved survival. Recently, consensus has developed that intensive follow-up with radiologic testing may lead to earlier detection of recurrence in some cases, but does not improve overall survival or quality of life (Consensus Conference, 1995). A randomized trial of 1,320 women treated for primary breast cancer compared clinical exam and annual mammography to clinical exam and annual mammography plus bone scans, liver sonograms, and chest X-rays at regular intervals (GIVIO Investigators, 1994). This study showed no difference in overall survival, time to detection of recurrence, or health-related quality of life between the two groups after a median follow-up of 71 months. Annual mammography is indicated to detect new primary cancers in the contralateral breast or recurrence in the ipsilateral breast after breast-conserving surgery (Consensus Conference, 1995) (Indicators 8 and 9). Periodic provider visits and clinical breast exam are indicated to detect signs and symptoms which would direct further diagnostic testing (Indicators 9 and 10).

REFERENCES

American College of Obstetricians and Gynecologists. 1991. Nonmalignant conditions of the breast. *ACOG Technical Bulletin* 156: 1-6.

American College of Obstetricians and Gynecologists. 1994. The role of the obstetrician-gynecologist in the diagnosis and treatment of breast disease. *ACOG Committee Opinion* 140: 1-2.

Bland KI, and Love N. 1992. Evaluation of common breast masses. *Postgraduate Medicine* 92 (5): 95-112.

Current Trials Working Party of the Cancer Research Campaign Breast Cancer Trials Group. Dec. 18 1996. Preliminary results from the cancer research campaign trial evaluating tamoxifen duration in women aged fifty years or older with breast cancer. *Journal of the National Cancer Institute* 88 (24) 1834-9.

Dixon JM, and Mansel RE. 1994. Symptom assessment and guidelines for referral. *British Medical Journal* 309 (17): 722-726.

Donegan WL. 1992. Evaluation of a palpable breast mass. *New England Journal of Medicine* 327 (13): 937-42.

Early Breast Cancer Trialists Collaborative Group (EBCTCG). 11 January 1992. Systemic treatment of early breast cancer by hormonal, cytotoxic, or immune therapy. Part II. *Lancet* 339 (8785): 71-85.

Early Breast Cancer Trialists Collaborative Group (EBCTCG). 4 January 1992. Systemic treatment of early breast cancer by hormonal, cytotoxic, or immune therapy. Part I. *Lancet* 339 (8784): 1-15.

GIVIO Investigators. 1994. Impact of follow-up testing on survival and health-related quality of life in breast cancer patients. A multicenter randomized controlled trial. *Journal of the American Medical Association* 271: 1587-1592.

Harris JR, Lippman ME, Veronesi U, and Willett W. 1992. Breast Cancer (First of Three Parts). *New England Journal of Medicine* 327 (5): 319-328.

Hortobagyi GN, and Buzdar AU. 1995. Current Status of Adjuvant Systemic Therapy for Primary Breast Cancer: Progress and Controversy. *CA Cancer a Journal for Clinicians* 45: 199-226.

MMWR. 1995. Consensus conference on follow-up of breast cancer patients. *Annals of Oncology* 6 (Suppl. 2): 69-70.

MMWR. 1996. Breast Cancer Incidence and Mortality - United States, 1992. *Morbidity and Mortality Weekly* 45 (39): 33-41.

National Institutes of Health. 18 June 1990. National Institutes of Health Consensus Development Conference on Treatment of Early-Stage Breast Cancer, National Institutes of Health.

US Preventative Services Task Force. 1996. *Guide to Clinical Preventative Services, 2nd ed.* Baltimore: Williams & Wilkins.

Winchester DP, and Cox JD. 1992. Standards for Breast Conservation Treatment. *CA Cancer:A Journal for Clinicians* 42 (3): 135-62.

RECOMMENDED QUALITY INDICATORS FOR BREAST CANCER DIAGNOSIS AND TREATMENT

The following criteria apply to women age 18 and older. Only the indicators in bold type were rated by this panel; the remaining indicators were endorsed by a prior panel.

Indicator	Quality of Evidence	Literature	Benefits	Comments
Diagnosis				
1. If a palpable breast mass has been detected, at least one of the following procedures should be completed within 3 months: • Fine needle aspiration; • Mammography; • Ultrasound; • Biopsy; • Follow-up visit.	III	ACOG, 1991; ACOG, 1994; Bland & Love, 1992; Dixon & Mansel, 1994	Reduce late-stage breast cancer. Decrease mortality from breast cancer.	Any breast mass may be an indicator of cancer and needs to be followed closely and/or investigated further. The 3-month time period is not specified in the literature but is probably generous. The modality of follow-up may differ depending on the patient and mass characteristics.
2. If a breast mass has been detected on two separate occasions, then either a biopsy, FNA or ultrasound should be performed within 3 months of the second visit.	III	ACOG, 1991; ACOG, 1994; Bland & Love, 1992; Dixon & Mansel, 1994	Reduce late-stage breast cancer. Decrease mortality from breast cancer.	A definite mass (as opposed to fibrocystic changes) needs further work-up. Although a follow-up visit to determine change in nature or size with menstrual cycle may be appropriate one time, a biopsy or FNA for diagnosis needs to occur if a definite mass is palpated twice. The time frame is debatable.
3. A biopsy or FNA should be performed within 6 weeks of either of the following circumstances: a. Mammography suggests malignancy;[1] b. Persistent palpable mass is not cystic on ultrasound.	III	ACOG, 1991	Reduce late-stage breast cancer. Decrease mortality from breast cancer.	Mammographic signs of malignancy or persistent solid mass require cytologic or histologic diagnosis to rule out malignancy.
4. A biopsy should be performed within 6 weeks if FNA cannot rule out malignancy.[2]	III	ACOG, 1994	Reduce late-stage breast cancer. Decrease mortality from breast cancer.	Histologic confirmation of the diagnosis is required if FNA of a solid mass is suspicious or non-diagnostic.

43

Treatment

Indicator	Quality of Evidence	Literature	Benefits	Comments
5. Women with Stage I or Stage II breast cancer should be offered a choice of modified radical mastectomy or breast-conserving surgery, unless contraindications to breast-conserving surgery[3] are present.	I	NIH, 1990; Winchester, 1992	Allow women the option of breast preservation while reducing mortality from breast cancer.	Breast-conserving surgery and modified radical mastectomy have equivalent survival outcomes.
6. Women treated with breast conserving surgery should begin radiation therapy within 6 weeks of completing either of the following (unless wound complications prevent the initiation of treatment): • last surgical procedure on the breast (including reconstructive surgery); or • chemotherapy, if patient receives adjuvant chemotherapy.	III	NIH, 1990; EBCTCG, 1992; Winchester, 1992	Reduce recurrence and mortality from breast cancer. Obtain maximum benefit from radiation therapy.	Although there may be a subset of women who do not benefit from radia- tion, current data do not allow identification of any subgroup in which radiation therapy can be avoided. Consensus states that radiation can begin as soon as the patient has healed adequately from the surgical procedure, usually within 2 to 4 weeks.
7. Women over age 50 with node-positive breast cancer should be treated with adjuvant systemic therapy to include one of the following: • Combination chemotherapy (more than one agent, lasting for at least 2 months); • Tamoxifen (20 mg/d for at least 2 years).	I	EBCTCG, 1992	Reduce recurrence and mortality from breast cancer.	Although adjuvant therapy has been shown to reduce recurrence and mortality in both node-positive and node-negative cases, the absolute risk of recurrence is smaller in node-negative cancer.

44

Follow-up

Indicator	Quality of Evidence	Literature	Benefits	Comments
8. Women with a history of breast cancer should have yearly mammography.	I	Consensus Conference, 1995; Givio, 1994	Detect recurrent or new primary breast cancers.	Yearly mammography and regular clinical exam have been shown to lead to equivalent survival and quality of life as more intensive follow-up programs.
9. Women diagnosed with breast cancer in the past 5 years should have a clinical breast exam in the past 6 months.	III	Winchester, 1992	Detect signs and symptoms of recurrence.	Signs and symptoms of recurrence detected during clinical exams should guide the use of ancillary diagnostic tests.
10. Women diagnosed with breast cancer more than 5 years ago should have a clinical breast exam in the past year.	III	Winchester, 1992	Detect signs and symptoms of recurrence.	Signs and symptoms of recurrence detected during clinical exams should guide the use of ancillary diagnostic tests.

Definitions and Examples

[1] Mammography suggests malignancy: Any mammogram in which the result reads "suggestive of malignancy, cannot rule out malignancy, or suspicious calcifications."

[2] FNA cannot rule out malignancy: Any pathology report except one which reads "fibroadenoma." This would include those that have insufficient tissue or normal breast tissue, because of the likelihood that the FNA may have missed the lesion.

[3] Contraindications to breast-conserving surgery: These include multicentric breast malignancies, large tumors relative to breast size, pathologic features of the tumor and certain collagen vascular diseases. Because of the subjective nature of this determination, any statement that breast conserving surgery is contraindicated will be accepted.

Quality of Evidence Codes

I	RCT
II-1	Nonrandomized controlled trials
II-2	Cohort or case analysis
II-3	Multiple time series
III	Opinions or descriptive studies

3. CERVICAL CANCER SCREENING[1]

Deidre Gifford, M.D.

This chapter is based primarily on the U.S. Preventive Services Task Forces (USPSTF) review of screening for cervical cancer (USPSTF, 1996) and the 1992 National Cancer Institute Workshop on management of abnormal cervical cytology (Kurman, 1994). In addition, we performed a MEDLINE search of English language literature between 1990 and 1996 using the search terms cervix dysplasia, cervix neoplasms, and vaginal smears. This document addresses the questions of which populations should be screened for cervical cancer and at what interval, as well as management of women with abnormal screening tests. This review does not address treatment of confirmed cervical cancer.

IMPORTANCE

There are approximately 16,000 new cases of cervical cancer diagnosed each year in the United States, and about 4,800 deaths annually from the disease (Wingo, 1995). The lifetime probability of dying from cervical cancer in the US is 0.3 percent (Ries, 1994). Five year survival for women with advanced (Stage IV) disease is about 14 percent, whereas it is about 90 percent for women with localized cancer (USPSTF, 1996). Cervical cancer is a good candidate for a screening program because it has a long preinvasive stage during which the disease can be detected and cured.

SCREENING

The Papanicolaou (Pap) smear is the primary method of screening for cervical cancer. Pap smears can detect early dysplastic cell changes which are precursors to invasive disease. Women in whom such abnormalities are detected can then have further diagnostic testing and treatment with

---

[1] This chapter is a revision of one written for an earlier project on quality of care for women and children (Q1). The expert panel for the current project was asked to review all of the indicators, but only rated new or revised indicators.

interventions such as colposcopy, biopsy, and cervical conization, which can prevent further progression of the disease.

Evidence of the effectiveness of screening programs comes from observational studies showing decreases in cervical cancer mortality following the introduction of population screening programs. Such decreases have been observed in the United States and Canada, as well as in several European countries (USPSTF, 1996). For example, data from Iceland demonstrated a rising cervical cancer mortality rate during the early 1960s. Screening was introduced in 1964, and by 1970 the annual mortality rate began to decline. By 1974, it had fallen significantly, decreasing from 23 per 100,000 in 1965-1969 to about 15 per 100,000 in 1970-74 (Johannesson et al., 1978). Further evidence comes from Canada, where the reduction in cervical cancer mortality has been noted to correlate with the proportion of the population screened with Pap tests (Eddy, 1990). In addition to this evidence, several case control studies have noted a marked decrease in risk of developing cervical cancer in women screened with pap smears when compared to unscreened women. Such studies indicate that screening for cervical cancer with Pap smears is highly effective, decreasing the occurrence of invasive cancer by 60 to 90 percent (Eddy, 1990).

The effectiveness of cervical cancer screening appears to increase with decreasing screening intervals. This evidence also comes from case control studies, which demonstrated decreased relative risks of invasive disease in women with shorter screening intervals (Eddy, 1990). However, there is also evidence that annual screening may produce only a minimally lower risk of invasive disease than screening every two to three years (USPSTF, 1996; Eddy, 1990). According to one study of eight cervical cancer screening programs in Europe and Canada, the incidence of cervical cancer can be reduced by 64 percent with a screening interval of ten years, by 84 percent with a five year interval, and by 91 percent, 93 percent and 94 percent with intervals of three, two and one years, respectively (IARC Working Group, 1986).

Several important risk factors have been identified for cervical cancer (Eddy, 1990). These include:

1. Race/ethnicity, with African Americans and Hispanics having a two-fold increased risk;

2. Early age at first sexual intercourse;

3. Multiple sexual partners;

4. Smoking;

5. Human immunodeficiency virus (HIV) infection; and

6. Human papillomavirus (HPV) infection.

There has been debate in the literature about whether or not women with such risk factors should be screened more frequently than the general population of women. Published recommendations leave room for physician discretion in screening such women. Consensus has been reached by the American Cancer Society, the National Cancer Institute, the American College of Obstetricians and Gynecologists (ACOG), the American Medical Association, the American Nurses Association, the American Academy of Family Physicians and the American Medical Womens Association (American Cancer Society, 1993; ACOG, 1995) on a guideline that recommends annual Pap smears for all women who are or have been sexually active, or who are at least 18 years of age. After three normal annual smears, and *if recommended by the physician*, less frequent testing is permitted. No upper age limit for cessation of testing is specified in this recommendation (Indicators 1, 2, 3 and 4).

The USPSTF (1996) makes similar recommendations about the onset of testing and adds that Pap tests should be performed at least every three years. The interval for each patient should be recommended by the physician based on risk factors (e.g., early onset of sexual intercourse, history of multiple sexual partners, low socioeconomic status). Women who have never been sexually active or who have had a total hysterectomy for benign indications with previously normal screening do not need regular Pap smears because they are not at risk for cervical cancer.

Some groups have proposed that women over the age of 65 who have had regular and normal screening prior to age 65 may not require further Pap screening because the incidence of disease is low in women this age with previously normal smears (Miller, 1991). The USPSTF states there is insufficient evidence to recommend an appropriate upper age limit for screening, but suggests that recommendations can be made on other grounds to discontinue regular testing after age 65 in women who have had regular previous screenings in which the smears have been consistently normal. They also state that women who have not had regular screening before the age of 65 should continue to receive smears every three years. (USPSTF, 1996). The ACOG does not support cessation of screening at any age, regardless of prior screening history (ACOG, 1995). It appears that the age at which screening for cervical cancer can safely be stopped, if any, is not clearly known.

Management Of Women With Abnormal Pap Smears

Although there is generally less consensus about appropriate treatment and follow-up of abnormal pap smears than there is about their effectiveness as a screening technique, reductions in cervical cancer mortality are dependent on follow-up and treatment of women who have positive screening exams. The classification of abnormal smears is variable, with different systems for reporting abnormalities (Table 3.1).

Table 3.1
Cytopathology Reporting Systems for Pap Smears

Class System	World Health Organization System	Cervical Intraepithelial Neoplasia System	The Bethesda System
I	Normal	Normal	Within normal limits

II	Inflammation		Other
			    Infection
			    Reactive and reparative

III	Dysplasia:
	    Mild
	    Moderate
	    Severe
		CIN-1
		CIN-2
			Squamous intraepithelial lesions:
			    Low grade
			    High grade

IV	Carcinoma in situ	CIN-3	
V	Invasive squamous cell carcinoma Adenocarcinoma	Invasive squamous cell carcinoma Adenocarcinoma	Squamous cell carcinoma Adenocarcinoma

Source: Miller et al., 1992

The Bethesda system was introduced to replace the previous Pap classifications and to facilitate precise communication between cytopathologists and clinicians. There is not universal agreement that it is superior to the CIN designations (Kurman et al., 1991). The Bethesda system contains a new classification, atypical squamous or glandular cells of undetermined significance or ASCUS (AGCUS). This category can be used by pathologists to signify the presence of atypical cells which are not clearly dysplastic but are of undetermined significance. The National Cancer Institute recommendations for follow-up of Pap smear abnormalities use the Bethesda Classification, and we have used the Bethesda Classification in recommending follow-up of mildly abnormal Pap smears. Recommendations for follow-up of abnormal smears have been summarized by the report of a Canadian National workshop on screening for cancer of the cervix (Miller, 1991), and a National Cancer Institute Workshop on management of abnormal cervical cytology (Kurman, 1994). First, they stress that screening recommendations (as summarized above) apply only to women with normal screening exams, and that women with abnormal smears should be screened and treated differently (Indicator 4). The National Cancer Institute Workshop recommends that women with low grade squamous intraepithelial lesions (LGSIL), which includes changes consistent with HPV infection without dysplasia, or atypical squamous cells of undetermined significance (ASCUS), should be rescreened at intervals of 6 to 12 months and referred for colposcopy if the abnormality persists at 24 months past the original smear (Indicators 6 and 7). The Canadian Consensus does not use the Bethesda system, but agrees with this management for atypia, mild dysplasia, CIN I, or HPV using the older designations. This management is based on the finding that many of these lesions will regress spontaneously without intervention (Montz et al., 1992); however, some have argued that the inconvenience, distress, and possibly the cost of this strategy are excessive, and that all women with abnormal smears should be referred immediately for colposcopic evaluation (Soutter, 1992; Wright, 1995). ACOG suggests that women with these low grade lesions may either be followed at six-month intervals or referred for colposcopy. All groups recommend colposcopic evaluation eventually for all women with persistent lesions (ACOG, 1993; Miller, 1991; Kurman, 1994) (Indicator 7).

There is agreement about follow-up of women with more dysplastic lesions on Pap smear. Women with Pap smears read as moderate dysplasia, severe dysplasia, carcinoma in-situ, CIN II or greater, high grade squamous intraepithelial lesions, squamous cell carcinoma or adenocarcinoma should be referred for colposcopic evaluation (Indicator 5). The prevention of cervical cancer is dependent on the diagnostic evaluation and treatment given to women with these abnormalities.

REFERENCES

American Cancer Society. 1993. *Guidelines for Cancer-Related Check-ups: an update*. American Cancer Society, Atlanta.

American College of Obstetricians and Gynecologists. August 1993. Cervical cytology: Evaluation and management of abnormalities. *ACOG Technical Bulletin* 183: 1-8.

American College of Obstetricians and Gynecologists. March 1995. Recommendations on Frequency of Pap Test Screening. *ACOG Committee Opinion* 152.

Eddy DM. 1990. Screening for cervical cancer. *Archives of Internal Medicine* 113 (3): 214-26.

IARC Working Group on Evaluation of Cervical Cancer Screening Programmes. 13 September 1986. Screening for squamous cervical cancer: Duration of low risk after negative results of cervical cytology and its implication for screening policies. *British Medical Journal* 293: 659-64.

Johannesson G, G Geirsson, and N Day. 1978. The effect of mass screening in Iceland, 1965-74, on the incidence and mortality of cervical carcinoma. *International Journal of Cancer* 21: 418-25.

Kurman RJ, et al. 15 June 1994. Interim Guidelines for Management of Abnormal Cervical Cytology. *Journal of the American Medical Association* 271 (23): 1866-69.

Kurman RJ, GD Malkasian, A Sedlis, et al. May 1991. From Papanicolaou to Bethesda: The rationale for a new cervical cytologic classification. *Obstetrics and Gynecology* 77 (5): 779-82.

Miller AB, G Anderson, J Brisson, et al. 15 November 1991. Report of a national workshop on screening for cancer for the cervix. *Canadian Medical Association Journal* 145 (10): 1301-25.

Montz FJ, Bradley J, Monk BJ, et al. September 1992. Natural History of the Minimally Abnormal Papanicolaou Smear. *Obstetrics and Gynecology* 80 (3): 385-88.

Richart RM, and Wright TC. 1993. Controversies in the management of low grade cervical intraepithelial neoplasia. *Cancer* 71: 1413-21.

Ries LAG, Miller BA, Hankey BF, et al. 1994. *SEER Cancer Statistics Review 1973-1991*. National Cancer Institute.

Souter WP. 23 May 1992. Conservative treatment of mild/moderate cervical dyskaryosis. *Lancet* 339: 1293.

US Preventative Services Task Force. 1996. *Guide to Clinical Preventative Services, 2nd ed*. Baltimore: Williams & Wilkins.

Wingo PA, Tong T, and Bolden S. 1995. Cancer Statistics 1995. *CA Cancer a Journal for Clinicians* 45: 8-30.

RECOMMENDED QUALITY INDICATORS FOR CERVICAL CANCER SCREENING

The following criteria apply to women age 18 and over. These indicators were not rated by this panel; they were endorsed by a prior panel.

	Indicator	Quality of Evidence	Literature	Benefits	Comments
1.	The medical record should contain the date and result of the last Pap smear.	II-2	USPSTF, 1996; ACOG, 1995; ACOG, 1993	Prevent cervical cancer morbidity and mortality.[1] Prevent cervical cancer.	The appropriate timing of the next Pap smear is determined by the time elapsed since the last smear, and the result of the last smear.
2.	Women who have not had a Pap smear within the last 3 years should have one performed (unless never sexually active with men or have had a hysterectomy for benign indications).	II-2	USPSTF, 1996; ACOG, 1995; ACOG, 1993	Prevent cervical cancer morbidity and mortality.[1] Prevent cervical cancer.	The maximum interval for women with intact uteri is every three years. The incidence of cervical cancer is increased when screening intervals exceed 3 years.
3.	Women who have not had 3 consecutive normal smears and who have not had a Pap smear within the last year should have one performed.	III	ACOG, 1995; ACS, 1993	Prevent cervical cancer morbidity and mortality.[1] Prevent cervical cancer.	A normal Pap smear is defined as one without atypia, dysplasia, CIS or invasive carcinoma. If there is no documentation of the actual pathology/cytology reports (e.g., because previous Pap smears were done at another facility) but there is documentation in the history that all previous Paps were normal, then the appropriate screening interval may be regarded as three years.
4.	Women with a history of cervical dysplasia or carcinoma-in-situ who have not had a Pap smear within the last year should have one performed.	III	Miller et al., 1991; ACOG, 1993	Prevent cervical cancer morbidity and mortality.[1] Prevent cervical cancer.	These women are at increased risk for cervical disease, and should not be returned to the usual screening intervals.
5.	Women with a severely abnormal Pap smear should have colposcopy performed within 3 months of the Pap smear date.[2]	III	Miller et al., 1991; Kurman, 1994	Prevent cervical cancer morbidity and mortality.[1]	Appropriate follow-up for abnormal findings is key in preventing progression to cervical cancer. The 3 month time period is arbitrary.

54

Indicator	Quality of Evidence	Literature	Benefits	Comments
6. If a woman has a Pap smear that shows a low grade lesion (ASCUS or LGSIL), then one of the following should occur within 6 months of the initial Pap: 1) repeat Pap smear; or 2) colposcopy.	III	Kurman, 1994	Prevent cervical cancer morbidity and mortality.[1]	Patients with these intermediate findings should be monitored closely. In many cases, abnormal findings resolve spontaneously, so follow-up with Pap smears or immediate colposcopy are both appropriate.
7. Women with a Pap smear that shows ASCUS or LGSIL, and who have had the abnormality documented on at least 2 Pap smears in a 2 year period should have colposcopy performed.	III	Kurman, 1994; ACOG, 1993	Prevent cervical cancer morbidity and mortality.[1]	Patients with intermediate findings should be monitored closely since some portion of these may represent preinvasive disease, or progress to a high-grade SIL. If findings persist, colposcopy should be performed. This may be difficult to operationalize for women who have not been enrolled in the same plan for two years or more.

Definitions and Examples

[1] Morbidity of cervical cancer includes postsurgical and chemotherapeutic complications, infertility, incontinence, and pain from metastases.
[2] Severely abnormal Pap smear: moderate dysplasia, severe dysplasia, carcinoma in situ, CIS, CIN II, CIN III, high grade SIL, squamous cell carcinoma, or adenocarcinoma.

Quality of Evidence Codes

I   RCT
II-1   Nonrandomized controlled trials
II-2   Cohort or case analysis
II-3   Multiple time series
III   Opinions or descriptive studies

55

4. COLORECTAL CANCER SCREENING

Patricia Bellas, M.D.

For this chapter, we reviewed the recently published clinical guidelines for colorectal cancer screening, prepared by an AHCPR/American Gastroenterological Association expert panel (AGA Guidelines, 1997). In addition, we reviewed the chapter on colorectal cancer screening in the second edition of the USPSTF Guide to Clinical Preventive Services (1996). Other review articles on this subject published between 1993 and 1996 were obtained using a MELVYL search (Van Dam, 1995; Ferrante, 1996; Cohen, 1996). When appropriate, original studies were reviewed (Winawer, 1993; Mandel, 1993; Selby, 1992; Muller, 1995; Newcomb, 1992; Bond, 1993; Kewenter, 1994; Ahlquist, 1993). In addition, we reviewed the chapter on laboratory screening tests in Health Promotion and Disease Prevention in Clinical Practice (Woolf, 1996). Recently published articles were identified from other unpublished reviews (Hardcastle, 1996; Kronborg, 1996; Allison, 1996; Rex, 1996; Read, 1997). Indicators for diagnosis, treatment, and follow-up of colorectal cancer can be found in Chapter 5.

IMPORTANCE

Colorectal cancer (CRC) is the third most commonly diagnosed cancer with an annual incidence of about 140,000. It is the second most common cause of cancer deaths, with about 55,000 deaths each year. Incidence increases significantly after age 50 and rises with age. Estimated five year survival is 91 percent for localized disease, 60 percent with regional spread, and six percent with distant metastasis. Unfortunately, 60 percent of patients with CRC already have regional or distant spread at the time of diagnosis (USPSTF, 1996). Racial differences in survival have been documented, with lower relative survival rates for African Americans than for whites.

SCREENING

Risk Factors

Persons considered at average risk for CRC comprise 75 percent of those with incident cancers. Those with one or more first degree relatives with CRC comprise 15 to 20 percent of all annual incident CRCs and have about twice the risk of a person with no such family history. This increased risk begins at a younger age, particularly if the family member's cancer occurred before age 55. For this reason, screening is recommended to begin at age 40 for individuals with a first degree relative with CRC (AGA Guidelines, 1997) (Indicator 1).

Rarer genetic syndromes -- familial adenomatous polyposis (FAP) and hereditary nonpolyposis colon cancer (HNPCC) -- confer a significantly increased risk of developing CRC. Patients with FAP have nearly a 100 percent risk of developing CRC by age 40. Genetic testing may be helpful, but endoscopy is usually necessary to determine gene expression; surveillance is not feasible, and the only preventive measure available is colectomy. Patients with FAP should have specialty consultation. CRC and adenomatous polyps develop at an earlier age and may progress more rapidly in patients with HNPCC (usually defined by family history, but also determined by genetic testing). Therefore, close surveillance is recommended as early as ages 20 to 30. In cases of uncertainty of diagnosis and long term management issues, specialty referral is usually appropriate. Persons with inflammatory bowel disease have an increased risk of CRC that is related to the extent and duration of disease. Persons with these genetic syndromes or inflammatory bowel disease should be made aware of their risks and options for therapy and/or surveillance (Indicator 2).

Evidence for Early Detection

There is *indirect* evidence that most CRCs develop from adenomatous polyps. Generally the sequence from small polyp to cancer is felt to occur over a time frame of ten to 15 years. A relatively small percent of adenomatous polyps (estimated at 2.5 per 1000 annually) actually progress to cancer. Adenomatous (neoplastic) polyps, which are usually considered premalignant, comprise one-half to two-thirds of colorectal polyps. Benign mucosal polyps or small benign hyperplastic polyps (<0.5 cm) comprise most of the rest (20 to 50 percent). Other histologic types are uncommon. Polyp characteristics associated with an increased risk of cancer include size >= 1 cm and tubulovillous or villous histology (AGA Guidelines, 1997). Studies suggest that less than one percent of adenomatous polyps under 1 cm are malignant and that small (<0.5 cm) tubular or hyperplastic polyps do not seem to be associated with any increase in risk for CRC.

Evidence to support aggressive polyp treatment is not strong. Perhaps the best evidence comes from the National Polyp Study (Winawer, 1993c). This study found a reduction in expected CRC incidence in those patients who underwent surveillance colonoscopy and removal of polyps, as compared with three different reference groups; suggesting that CRC can be prevented by colonoscopic polypectomy. Additional but weaker evidence is offered by two case-control VA studies by Muller and Sonnenberg (1995a, 1995b); one compared 8722 colon cancer and 7629 rectal cancer patients to matched controls. The influence of having had an endoscopic examination of the colon on the development of colorectal cancer was tested by conditional multiple logistic regression analysis. These procedures (flexible sigmoidoscopy, colonoscopy and polypectomy) reduced the risk of developing CRC by 50 percent (colon cancer: OR 0.51, CI 0.44-0.58; rectal cancer: OR 0.55, CI 0.47-0.64) and this protective influence appeared to last six years (Muller and Sonnenberg, 1995a). The other study compared 4411 veterans who died of CRC with controls. Any diagnostic colon procedure was associated with a decrease in mortality from CRC (OR 0.67, CI 0.54-0.82), with the greatest risk reduction associated with tissue removal, through biopsy, fulguration, or polypectomy (OR 0.41-0.43)(Muller and Sonnenberg, 1995b). Population trends do show a decrease in both CRC incidence and mortality since the mid 1980s. To what extent identification and removal of premalignant polyps have contributed to this trend remains speculative.

The American College of Gastroenterology undertook a review in 1993 to outline the preferable approach to management of polyps in patients with nonfamilial colorectal polyps (Bond, 1993). In 1997, the American Gastroenterological Association expert panel published clinical guidelines for colorectal cancer screening (AGA guidelines, 1997). If large polyps (>1 cm) are found on sigmoidoscopy or barium enema, the patient should be recommended to have colonoscopy to remove these polyps and evaluate the rest of the colon for additional lesions (Indicator 3). In addition, polyps <1 cm should be biopsied (Indicator 4). At colonoscopy, most polyps are removed. A total excisional biopsy is preferred so the entire polyp can be examined histologically. Small sessile polyps are usually examined by biopsy and fulgurated, as are most small polyps (<5 cm). When numerous small lesions are found, representative biopsies are recommended prior to fulguration. Large sessile polyps (>= 2cm) may be difficult to remove and tend to recur. Because these types of polyps are felt to have an increased malignant potential, follow-up colonoscopy every three to six months is necessary until completeness of excision is documented (Bond, 1993).

Post-polypectomy surveillance needs to be individualized according to the age and comorbidity of the patient. Most should have an exam at three years to look for missed synchronous and metachronous adenomas (Zauber, 1997). Persons with a single tubular adenoma under 1 cm may not need follow-up. Generally, if the first follow-up exam is negative, the surveillance interval can be increased to five years. There is good evidence from a randomized controlled trial (Winawer, 1993b) that an initial follow-up exam at one year offers no benefit over an exam at three years; therefore our indicator reflects the longer time period (Indicator 5).

Woolf (1996), in his book "Health Promotion and Disease Prevention in Clinical Practice," clearly describes the documentation needed to facilitate appropriate follow-up for endoscopic procedures. The polyp guidelines do not explicitly discuss procedure documentation; however, adequate documentation is essential to inform future management (Indicator 6).

Efforts have been made to define the relationship of polyp distribution in the colon. Evidence exists that patients with adenomatous polyps found in the rectosigmoid area have a one in three chance of having additional adenomas in the proximal colon. Characteristics of proximal adenomas (greater than 1 cm and histology) seem to correlate with distal lesions; therefore, our recommended quality indicator states that positive findings on sigmoidoscopy should be followed by colonoscopy to remove polyps and to look for synchronous lesions in the rest of the colon (Indicator 7). According to the AGA Guidelines (1997), a "positive" screening sigmoidoscopy exam is the finding of either a cancer, or a polyp greater than 1 cm. There is no consensus regarding the significance of polyps less than 1 cm, although many experts

60

also recommend colonoscopy for patients who have polyps between 0.6 and 1 cm (Bond, 1993). In a recently published prospective study by Read (1997) evaluating the significance of polyps detected by sigmoidoscopy, the size of the index adenoma found on sigmoidoscopy did not correlate with the prevalence of proximal neoplasia. Twenty-nine percent of those with polyps under 5 mm had proximal lesions, but the size of the index adenomas did correlate with the finding of advanced proximal neoplasia.

Effectiveness of Screening Tests

Fecal Occult Blood Test (FOBT)

Standard FOBT consists of testing two samples from each of three consecutive stools for the presence of fecal occult blood. Most tests are qualitative, based on a guaiac-based test for peroxidase activity (hemoccult). These tests are based on the fact that colorectal cancers tend to bleed more than normal mucosa. Very large polyps may bleed, whereas small ones are unlikely to do so. False positive results can occur from dietary sources and from upper gastrointestinal bleeding, often associated with gastric irritants such as aspirin or other non-steroidal anti-inflammatory drugs (NSAIDS). False negative tests can occur due to the intermittent nature of bleeding from CRCs or polyps, dietary ingestion of antioxidants, and extended delay in testing the samples (dehydration of the slides). Sensitivity may vary from 26 to 92 percent and specificity from 99 to 90 percent. Rehydration of slides prior to testing does improve sensitivity, but with a loss of specificity and resultant drop in positive predictive value from six to two percent. Quantitative testing (HemoQuant) has not clearly been demonstrated to offer an advantage over other testing (USPSTF, 1996). The wide range of reported sensitivity and specificity is due to multiple factors including study design, type of test and number of specimens collected, and adherence to dietary restrictions. These factors make it difficult to directly compare test performance. Newer (and more expensive) tests based on hemoglobin immunoassays (HemeSelect) may improve the performance of these tests, and strategies using two stage testing seem to show more acceptable sensitivity and specificity (HemeSensa followed by HemeSelect) (Allison, 1996).

When FOBT is performed on asymptomatic persons, the majority of positive reactions are falsely positive for neoplasia, resulting in a large number of persons subsequently receiving diagnostic testing such as colonoscopy or barium enema. In large studies, FOBT positivity ranges from 1.1 to 6.2 percent averaging three percent (Van Dam, 1996).

Four controlled trials (three randomized and one unrandomized) have looked at FOBT screening and mortality from CRC (see Table 4.1). In most cases a positive FOBT is defined as one or more positive square. In all studies, full examination of the colon by colonscopy or DCBE was offered. In the Nottingham study (Hardcastle et al., 1996), if only one to four squares reacted the FOBT was repeated with dietary restriction. Only persons with positive initial tests of five or more squares or repeat positive tests were further studied.

The Minnesota colon cancer trial (Mandel, 1993) randomized 46,551 clinic patients (volunteers) aged 50 to 80 to receive either annual FOBT, biennial FOBT or usual care. All positive FOBTs were followed by colonoscopy. After 13 years of follow-up, there was a 33 percent reduction in cumulative CRC mortality in the annually screened group compared to the control (usual care) group. A lesser reduction in CRC mortality found in the biennially screened group was not statistically significant. The detection and removal of adenomatous polyps in the screened group did not appear to contribute to the reduction in mortality or prevalence of CRC. Almost one-third of the study participants ended-up receiving diagnostic testing because of a positive FOBT. Critics have suggested that the mortality reduction observed may be due to the large number of colonoscopies performed independent of any benefit from FOBT. Some have attributed one-third to one-half of the mortality reduction to the large number of colonoscopies performed.

The Memorial Sloan-Kettering Cancer Center - Strang Clinic trial (Winawer, 1993a) was a controlled study comparing sigmoidoscopy alone versus sigmoidoscopy plus FOBT. Twenty thousand patients over age 40 who attended this preventive medicine clinic were evaluated in two different study and control groups. Non-rehydrated slides were used. If a positive result was obtained, the patient was referred for DCBE and colonoscopy. All patients additionally received a flexible sigmoidoscopy, and any with polyps over 3 mm were referred for full colonoscopy. After ten years the CRC mortality rate was lower (0.36 versus 0.63) in the study group for trial II (n=11,479); however it was of borderline statistical significance. Most of the benefit was found in the initial screening (finding prevalent cases of cancer). Problems with this study included the fact that some of the patients had symptoms and compliance with follow-up screening was very low.

Two large European trials (Nottingham and Danish) have investigated the effect of FOBT screening on mortality. The Nottingham study (Hardcastle, 1996) randomized 150,251 patients aged 45 to 74 to be offered FOBT every two years (nonrehydrated). After a mean follow-up of 7.8 years, there was a reduction in CRC mortality of 15 percent (OR 0.85; CI 0.74-0.98). In the Danish study, 61,993 people aged 45 to 75 were randomized to be offered FOBT every two years. After ten years of follow-up, there was an 18 percent reduction in mortality from CRC (OR 0.82; CI 0.68-0.99) (Kronborg, 1996).

The main concerns regarding FOBT relate to the risks associated with subsequent diagnostic tests following positive screening, and, given the low sensitivity and specificity of the FOBT, the number of diagnostic work-ups performed. There are also concerns regarding the interpretation of a false negative test. Compliance with FOBT has varied over many of the studies, but ranges from 30 to 90 percent (AGA Guidelines, 1997). Although there is some evidence that annual testing may have greater benefit (Mandel, 1993), based on the two European population trials which used biennial screening, our indicator requires that FOBT testing be offered within a two year period to all average risk patients over 50 unless another screening method is used (Indicator 10). Testing need not be continued after age 80. If a test is positive, the patient should be notified and offered a diagnostic colon evaluation (colonoscopy or double contrast barium enema [DCBE] with or without flexible sigmoidoscopy) within a six month period of time (Ransohoff, 1997) (Indicator 8) (see Table 4.1).

A FOBT need not be offered if one of the other tests have been performed. However, if a patient is unwilling to have one of the other tests done for screening purposes, they should be offered the option of a FOBT after appropriate counseling regarding diagnostic evaluation of positive tests (Indicator 9).

Sigmoidoscopy

Three types of scopes have been used in screening: a 25 cm rigid scope, and 30 cm or 60 cm flexible scopes. Endoscopic examination detects nearly all lesions greater than 1 cm and 70 to 80 percent of polyps less than 1 cm, if

those lesions are within the reach of the scope. Data based on distribution
of lesions within the colon suggest that the 60 cm scope should be able to
detect 40 to 60 percent of CRC cancers and polyps; the 35 cm scope can detect
30 to 40 percent of the lesions: the rigid 25 cm scope can reach 20 to 30
percent of the lesions (AGA Guidelines, 1997).

There are several case control studies and several follow-up studies that
address sigmoidoscopic screening. The Kaiser study (Selby, 1992) compared
patients who died of CRC with age and sex matched controls. They found a 59
percent reduction in mortality (OR 0.41, CI 0.25-0.69) from cancers within
reach of the rigid sigmoidoscope. This protective effect, which was not
present for more proximal cancers, appeared to be present for nine to ten
years. In a smaller case control study by Newcomb, patients who had undergone
one or more sigmoidoscopic exam had an 80 percent reduction in the risk of
death from rectosigmoid cancer compared to those who did not (OR 0.21, CI
0.08-0.52). A third study is the previously mentioned VA study (Muller and
Sonnenberg, 1995). In this study, the protective effect appeared to last six
years. Our indicator requires a screening interval of five years as
recommended by the AGA guidelines, although there is no additional evidence to
support this (Indicator 10). As noted earlier, all significant findings on
sigmoidoscopy should be evaluated with colonoscopy (Indicator 7).

Complications from sigmoidoscopy are uncommon; a low level of perforation
(one to two per 10,000) has been reported. Other criticisms of this method
include the fact that proximal lesions may exist beyond the reach of the scope
without the presence of distal lesions. Some have suggested combining
sigmoidoscopy with FOBT, however there is not enough evidence to recommend for
or against this method of screening.

Colonoscopy

Colonoscopy is a much more costly procedure and usually requires
sedation. Ideally, the total colon should be visualized, and this happens
about 80 to 95 percent of the time. There are no published studies examining
the effectiveness of *screening* colonoscopy in reducing CRC mortality.
Indirect evidence of its effectiveness is based on two facts: (1) detecting
and removing polyps appears to reduce the incidence of CRC (Winawer, 1993c;
Muller, 1995a; Muller, 1995b); (2) detecting cancer early lowers mortality

from the disease and colonoscopy is able to detect most of these lesions. The trials for FOBT have also included colonoscopy as part of the intervention.

Complications of colonoscopy are more common than with any of the other screening tests. The average reported risk of perforation is one per 1000, major hemorrhage in three per 1000 and complication deaths in one to three per 10,000. There is limited evidence on how often to screen; a study by Rex (1996) reported no significant findings during repeat colonoscopy done five years after an inital negative colonoscopy. Based on indirect findings (i.e., presumed length of time for development of CRC, duration of protective effect in case-control studies), the AGA Guidelines panel found screening colonoscopy every ten years to be adequate (Indicator 10). Given concerns of possible complications and expense, our proposed quality indicator states that colonoscopy screening should not be repeated in less than five years provided the previous colonoscopy was negative (Indicator 11).

Barium Enema

Barium enema can image the entire colon in most examinations, with about five to ten percent of tests being unsatisfactory. Double contrast barium enema (DCBE) is the preferred test. Studies suggest that the sensitivity of DCBE (usually the gold standard is colonoscopy) is 50 to 80 percent for polyps under 1 cm, 70 to 90 percent for polyps over 1 cm, and 55 to 85 percent for early cancers (AGA Guidelines, 1997). The specificity is 90 percent (USPSTF, 1996). DCBE may not be as effective at detecting lesions in the rectal area, therefore some recommend also performing flexible sigmoidoscopy; the combination of DCBE and flexible sigmoidoscopy has a sensitivity of 98 percent for cancers, and 99 percent for adenomas.

There is only indirect evidence to support the effectiveness of using barium enema in screening. There is evidence from previously mentioned studies that detecting polyps and early cancers by other types of screening tests reduces the incidence and mortality from CRC and DCBE has the capability of detecting many of these same lesions. The most serious potential complication of barium enema is perforation; however, there is not enough information published in the literature to determine how often this happens. It is felt to be safer than colonoscopy. Since significant findings on DCBE need to be further evaluated with diagnostic or therapeutic colonoscopy, leading to further expense, some have argued that colonoscopy should be the preferred test.

Computer Modeling

The AHCPR/AGA expert panel evaluated the various screening tests for CRC using computer modeling. The results of this effort are summarized in Table 4.2. According to these data, all of the screening strategies were more effective in saving lives than no screening, and the number of years of life saved are similar across screening strategies.

Screening Strategies

There are several options for individual patients and physicians to choose in regards to screening strategies. These include annual FOBT, screening flexible sigmoidoscopy every five years, combined FOBT and flexible sigmoidoscopy, DCBE every five to ten years, or colonoscopy every ten years. Limitations to any one strategy may include false positives, false negatives, high cost, unacceptability to the patient, unavailability of the test, and the risk of complications (Leard, 1997). All patients should have risks and benefits of these screening procedures explained to them, and a history of previously performed colon tests should be documented to avoid unnecessary repetition of tests. The AGA Guidelines have been endorsed by the American Cancer Society, American College of Gastroenterology, American Gastroenterological Association, American Society of Colon and Rectal Surgeons, and the American Society for Gastrointestinal Endoscopy. The USPSTF also recommended screening with either FOBT or sigmoidoscopy and gave this a "B" recommendation.

Risk stratification is important in determining which patients may benefit from other screening strategies recommended to them. It is important to inquire and document family history of CRCs and personal history of polyps or previous negative screens to limit screening test risks. However, there is no direct evidence that surveillance will reduce mortality in these high risk populations.

Table 4.1

Clinical Trials of Fecal Occult Blood Tests

	University of Minnesota (Mandell)	Sloan-Kettering Strang Clinic (Winawer)	Swedish Study (Kewenter)	Nottinham study (Hardcastle)	Danish Study (Kronborg)
Year begun	1975	1975	1982	1984	1985
Number of Subjects	46,000	2 groups of 10,000 each	68,308 (3 cohorts)	107,000	62,000
Randomized	YES	NO	YES	YES	YES
Type of setting	volunteers	preventive medicine clinic	population based	population based	population based
Age of enrollees	50-80	>40	60-64	50-75	45-74
Method	Rehydrated (3 cards, 2 slides each)	Non-rehydrated, 3 cards; both groups also received sigmoidoscopy	Initial non-rehydrated, subsequent rehydrated	Non-rehydrated	Non-rehydrated
Frequency	Annual and biennial	Annual	Repeated x1 @16-22 months	Biennial	Biennial
Compliance with FOBT	77%	74% first round	63% initial 60% on rescreen	59.6%(at least 1 round of screening)	67%
Definition of a positive test	1 or more slides reacting	1 or more slides reacting	1 cohort offered diagnostic work-up only if repeat test was positive. Number of slides not discussed	5 or 6 slides reacting on first test or 1 slide positive on repeat	1 or more slides reacting

Table 4.1

Clinical Trials of Fecal Occult Blood Tests
(continued)

	University of Minnesota (Mandell)	Sloan-Kettering Strang Clinic (Winawer)	Swedish Study (Kewenter)	Nottinham Study (Hardcastle)	Danish Study (Kronborg)
% Positive	9.8%	Trial 1 = 1.4% Trial 2 = 2.6% (for 1st test)	Non-rehydrated=1.9% rehydrated = 5.8-14.3% retest=2.3-4.6%	2.3%	1.1%
Sensitivity	49.5	70	79.4	74	48
Specificity	90.4	98	91.8	98	99
PPV for CRC	2.2%	17% inital less subsequent	4.1%	12%	17% inital 9% final round
% receiving diagnostic tests	Annual: 38% Biennial: 28%	Unclear	3.8% first screen 5.1% rescreen	4%	4.3%
Total years of follow-up	13	9	7	8	10
CRC Mortality ratio (OR)	Annual: 0.67 (CI 0.50-0.87) Biennial: 0.94 (CI 0.68-1.31)	0.57 , CI not given, authors note borderline significance	Not reported	0.85 (CI 0.74-0.98)	0.82 (CI 0.68-0.99)
Decrease in overall deaths	No change	No change	Not reported	No change	No change
Decrease in CRC incidence	No	Not clear	No	No	No

Source: Adapted from Ferrante, 1996

Table 4.2

Computer model of clinical consequences of 100,000 people entering a program of screening for CRC at age 50 years and remaining in it until age 85 or death.

Screening Strategy	Annual FOBT	Sigmoid- oscopy every 5 years	FOBT + sigmoid- oscopy every 5 years	Ba enema every 5 years	Ba enema every 10 years	Ba enema + sigmoidoscopy every 5 years	Colono- scopy every 10 years
Number of Screening tests performed	2,703,041 FOBT	569,816	FOBT 2,704,501 Sigmoid 424,301	566,162	320,579	Ba Enema 568,223 Sigmoid 568,230	327,913
Consequences							
False positive screening tests	215,830	3897	218,964	26,346	13,857	30,985	1442
Diagnostic evaluations	226,295	14,996	231,627	73,711	52,963	74,214	N/A
Cancer cases	2610	3013	1901	-604	2176	1113	1418
Cancers detected	2422	568	1758	-285	1501	916	1095
Cancer deaths prevented	1330	967	1609	1663	1442	1889	1763
Complication deaths	52	9	58	34	24	46	73
Perforations	304	20	312	97	69	100	445
Major bleeding episodes	741	49	757	248	178	243	1075
Minor complications	767	49	772	259	181	249	1101
Years of life saved by screening	12,325	8328	11,760	12,568	11,035	14,655	12,904
(95% CI)	(±523)	(±500)	(±512)	(±506)	(±526)	(±526)	(±522)

Source: AGA guidelines 1997, Table 7, page 627.
NOTE: The number of cancers detected varies because polyp removal reduces the incidence of CRC, therefore, the more frequently polyps are removed the fewer cases of CRC occur to be detected. With no screening, the number of cancer cases expected is 4,988 and the number of cancer deaths is 2,391.

REFERENCES

AGA and AHCPR expert panel. 1997. Colorectal cancer screening: clinical guidelines and rational. *Gastroenterology* 112: 594-642.

Allison J, Tekawa I, Ransom L, and Adrain A. 1996. A Comparison of fecal occult-blood tests for colorectal-cancer screening. *New England Journal of Medicine* 334 (3): 155-159.

Bond JH. 1993. Polyp Guideline: diagnosis, treatment, and surveillance for patients with nonfamilial colorectal polyps. *Archives of Internal Medicine* 119: 836-843.

Bond JH. 1995. Evolving strategies for colonscopic management of patients with colorectal polyps. *Endoscopy* 27: 38-42.

Cohen L. 1996. Colorectal cancer: A primary care approach to screening. *Geriatrics* 51: 45-50.

Ferrante J. 1996. Colorectal cancer screening. *Medical Clinics of North America* 80 (1): 27-43.

Hardcastle J, et al. 1996. Randomised controlled trial of faecal-occult-blood screening for colorectal cancer. *Lancet* 348: 1472-77.

Kewenter H, et al. 1994. Results of screening, rescreening, and follow-up in a prospective randomized study for detection of colorectal cancer by fecal occult blood testing. *Scandanavian Journal of Gastroenterology* 29: 468-473.

Kronborg O, et al. 1996. Randomised study of screening for colorectal cancer with faecal-occult-blood test. *Lancet* 348: 1467-71.

Leard L, Savides T, and Ganiats T. 1997. Patient preferences for colorectal cancer screening. *Journal of Family Practice* 45 (3): 211-218.

Mandel J, et al. 1993. Reducing mortality from colorectal cancer by screening for fecal occult blood. (for the Minnesota Colon Cancer Control Study). *New England Journal of Medicine* 328: 1365-1371.

Muller A, and Sonnenberg A. 1995. Prevention of colorectal cancer by flexible endoscopy and polypectomy. *Archives of Internal Medicine* 123: 904-910.

Muller A, and Sonnenberg A. 1995. Protection by endoscopy against death from colorectal cancer. *Archives of Internal Medicine* 155: 1741-1748.

Newcomb P, et al. 1992. Screening Sigmoidoscopy and colorectal cancer mortality. *Journal of the National Cancer Institute* 84: 1572-1575.

Ransohoff D and Lang C. 1997. Screening for colorectal cancer with the fecal occult blood test: A background paper. *Annuals of Internal Medicine* 126: 811-822.

Ransohoff D and Lang C. 1997. Suggested technique for fecal occult blood testing and interpretation in colorectal cancer screening. *Archives of Internal Medicine* 126: 808-810.

Read T, Read J, and Butterly L. 1997. Importance of adenomas 5 mm or less in diameter that are detected by sigmoidoscopy. *New England Journal of Medicine* 336: 8-12.

Rex D, et al. 1996. 5-year incidence of adenomas after negative colonoscopy in asymptomatic average-risk persons. *Gastroenterology* 111: 1178-1181.

Selby J, et al. 1992. A case-control study of screening sigmoidoscopy and mortality from colorectal cancer. *New England Journal of Medicine* 326 (10): 653-7.

Selby J, et al. 1993. Effect of fecal occult blood testing on mortality from colorectal cancer. *Archives of Internal Medicine* 118: 1-6.

U.S. Preventive Services Task Force. 1996. *Guide to Clinical preventive services 2nd Edition*. Baltimore: Williams & Wilkins.

Van Dam J, Bond J, and Sivak M. 1995. Fecal occult blood screening for colorectal cancer. *Archives of Internal Medicine* 155: 2389-2402.

Winawer S, et al. 1993. Prevention of colorectal cancer by colonoscopic polypectomy. *New England Journal of Medicine* 329: 1977-81.

Winawer S, et al. 1993. Randomized comparison of surveillance intervals after colonoscopic removal of newly diagnosed adenomatous polyps. *New England Journal of Medicine* 328: 901-6.

Winawer S, et al. 1993. Screening for colorectal cancer with fecal occult blood testing and sigmoidoscopy. *Journal of the National Cancer Institute* 85: 1311-1318.

Woolf, S. 1996. *Laboratory screening tests*. Baltimore: Williams & Wilkins, 115-121.

Zauber A, and Winawer S. 1997. Initial management and follow-up surveillance of patients with colorectal adenomas. *Gastroenterology Clinics of North America* 26 (1): 85-101.

RECOMMENDED QUALITY INDICATORS FOR COLORECTAL CANCER SCREENING

The following criteria apply to men and women age 18 and older.

Indicator	Quality of Evidence	Literature	Benefits	Comments
Persons with elevated colon cancer risks				
1. Patients documented in the chart as having one or more first degree relatives with CRC should be offered at least one of the following colon cancer screening test beginning at age 40: • FOBT; • Sigmoidoscopy; • Colonoscopy; • DCBE.	I, II, III	AGA guidelines	Decrease CRC mortality and possibly reduce CRC morbidity.	Persons with a family history of CRC comprise 15-20% of incident CRCs. There is evidence that in the presence of a positive family history, the risk for CRC at age 40 approaches that of an average risk person aged 50. I - good evidence that screening can reduce CRC mortality. II - good epidemiological evidence that family history confers increased risk at an early age. III - expert opinion that these patients be screened at an early age.
2. The chart should document discussion of the risk of CRC and risks and benefits of surveillance/screening for all patients with elevated risk of CRC due to any of the following indications: a. Inflammatory bowel disease of at least 10 years duration; b. Familial adenomatous polyposis syndromes; c. Hereditary nonpolyposis colon cancer (HNPCC).	III	AGA guidelines; USPSTF, 1996	Decrease CRC mortality.	For inflammatory bowel disease, the risk of CRC is related to duration and extent of disease and needs to be individualized. Patients with familial polyposis syndromes need endoscopy to document phenotype; screening/surveillance is not beneficial and patients may choose colectomy. For patients with HNPCC colonoscopy is the preferred test; screening/surveillance needs to be performed at a much earlier age and more frequently.

Indicator	Quality of Evidence	Literature	Benefits	Comments
Average risk, asymptomatic persons[1]				
3. Providers should offer to remove all polyps with either of the following characteristics within 6 weeks of detection: a. size greater than 1 cm; b. adenomatous histology.	II-3 III	Winawer,1993; Bond, 1993; AGA guidelines, 1997	Decrease CRC risk.	Colonoscopic polypectomy resulted in a lower than expected incidence of CRC as compared with 3 referent groups (Winawer, 1993). Most experts accept that most CRCs arise from adenomas. It is recommended that all polyps be biopsied to determine histology.
4. All polyps found on screening sigmoidoscopy should be biopsied at that time.	III	AGA Guidelines 1997; Bond, 1993	Diagnose cancer; determine CRC risk and need for further studies.	Polyp histology is important to determine diagnosis and prognosis.
5. Surveillance colonoscopy should not be repeated sooner than 3 years following the of removal of adenomatous polyps in otherwise average risk patients.[2]	I	Winawer, 1993	Decrease risk of complications.	Follow-up examinations at one year showed no benefit over a three year follow-up, provided all initial polyps were successfully removed, and none were sessile polyps >2 cm.
6. Procedure note documentation for endoscopic management of polyps should include: a. whether biopsy only versus complete removal of polyps was performed; b. location of any polyps removed endoscopically; c. polyp type: sessile versus pedunculated.	III	Bond, 1993; Woolf,1996	Guide further management; possibly decrease CRC risk.	Woolf clearly describes appropriate documentation needed to facilitate appropriate follow-up. The polyp guidelines do not explicitly discuss procedure documentation, however, the information included in this indicator is needed to determine future management.
7. All patients with positive[3] screening sigmoidoscopy tests should be offered a diagnostic colonoscopy.	II-2, III	Selby,1992; Newcomb, 1992; Muller, 1995	Reduce CRC mortality risk.	Proximal synchronous neoplasia (cancer or polyps) are correlated with distal lesions. There is controversy for the follow-up of tubular adenomas < 1 cm.

73

Indicator	Quality of Evidence	Literature	Benefits	Comments
8. If a screening FOBT is positive,[4] a diagnostic evaluation of the colon[5] should be offered within a 6 month period.	I, III	Mandel, 1993; Winawer,1993; Hardcastle, 1996; Kronborg, 1996; AGA Guidelines 1997	Reduce CRC mortality and possibly reduce CRC morbidity.	All of the studies of FOBT included a diagnostic evaluation of the entire colon for positive tests. A 6 month time frame seems reasonable although there is no evidence to support this. The definition of a positive test is based on the AGA Guidelines recommendation for standard Hemoccult II; some studies used a different interpretation (see Table 4.1).
9. A FOBT should be offered to those who refuse other screening tests for CRC.	I	Mandel, 1993; Winawer,1993; Hardcastle, 1996; Kronborg, 1996	Decrease mortality from CRC and possibly reduce morbidity.	Some persons may not be willing to undergo colonoscopy or sigmoidoscopy or DCBE for screening purposes. There is good evidence that screening FOBT reduce CRC mortality.
10. All adults age 52 to 80 should be offered at least one of the following colon cancer screening tests: • FOBT[6] (if not done in the past 2 years); • Sigmoidoscopy (if not done in the past 5 years); • Colonoscopy (if not done in the past 10 years); • Double contrast barium enema (if not done in the past 5 years).	I, II-2 II-2, II-2, III III	Mandel, 1993; Winawer, 1993; Kronborg, 1996; Hardcastle, 1996; Selby, 1992; Newcomb ,1992; Muller, 1995; USPSTF, 1996, 1997 AGA Guidelines	Decrease mortality from CRC and possibly reduce CRC morbidity.	Three randomized trials show modest decreased mortality from CRC with FOBTs. Although recommendations and studies seem to support annual FOBT, population studies showing decreased CRC morbidity have only been shown with biennial testing. Three case control studies show a decrease CRC mortality risk with sigmoidoscopy. Indirect evidence supports colonoscopy and DCBE for screening. Indicator begins at age 52 so that all eligible patients will have been over 50 for at least 2 years.
11. Colonoscopy screening should not be done more frequently than every 5 years provided the previous colonoscopy was negative and procedure note specifies adequate exam.	II, III	Selby, 1992; Muller, 1995; AGA guidelines 1997; Winawer, 1993; Rex,1996	Decrease risk of complications.	If an adequate test was performed, studies support little benefit in rescreening at less than this interval.

Definitions and Examples

[1] These indicators do not apply to patients documented to have a life expectancy of less than 5 years.

[2] Persons without a familial colon cancer syndrome or inflammatory bowel disease or personnel history of CRC.

[3] A positive or significant finding on sigmoidoscopy includes: one or more polyps greater than 1 cm., any polyp with villous or tubulovillous histology, cancer.

[4] For a Hemoccult II test, a positive test is 1 or more cells reacting ; other types of FOBT may also be acceptable.

[5] Colonoscopy or DCBE (with or without sigmoidoscopy).

[6] Standard FOBT(peroxidase based) should consist of 2 samples from each of 3 consecutive stools (preferably following appropriate dietary instructions).

Quality of Evidence Codes

I   Randomized Controlled Trial (RCT)
II-1   Nonrandomized controlled trials
II-2   Cohort or case analysis
II-3   Multiple time series
III   Opinions or descriptive studies

5. COLORECTAL CANCER TREATMENT

Jennifer Lynn Reifel, MD

The core references for this chapter include the textbook *Cancer Treatment* (Haskell, 1995), CancerNet PDQ Information for Health Care Professionals on colon cancer and rectal cancer (CancerNet, 1997), and recent review articles (Nogueras and Jagelman, 1993; Staniunas and Schoetz, 1993; Stein and Coller, 1993; Moertel, 1994; Kemeny et al., 1993; Levitan, 1993). Recent review articles were selected from a MEDLINE search identifying all English language review articles published on colorectal cancer diagnosis and treatment since 1992. Where the core references cited studies to support individual indicators, they have been included in the references. Whenever possible, they have been supplemented with the results of randomized controlled trials.

IMPORTANCE

Colorectal cancer (adenocarcinoma) is the second most frequent cause of cancer mortality in the United States. It is estimated that 133,500 people will be diagnosed with colorectal cancer in 1996 and 54,900 will die from the disease (Parker et al., 1996).

In addition, colorectal cancer is curable in approximately 50 percent of patients when it is diagnosed and treated while still localized to the bowel and amenable to surgery.

SCREENING

The quality indicators for colorectal cancer screening and the treatment of benign polyps is covered in Chapter 4.

DIAGNOSIS

Patients with colorectal cancer may be asymptomatic at presentation. A patient with a positive fecal occult blood test or with a large (> 1 cm) or adenomatous polyp discovered on sigmoidoscopy should undergo a full colonoscopy to look for neoplasm and to excise any polyps (Winawer et al., 1997). The symptoms associated with colorectal carcinoma depend upon the size and location of the tumor. Tumors of the right colon, which contains fluid stool, tend to be larger on presentation and produce symptoms of abdominal pain, bleeding, and weight loss. As the left side of the colon contains semi-solid or solid stool, tumors there often cause obstructive symptoms, or a decrease in stool caliber, and may also be associated with bleeding. Patients over age 50 who present with the above symptoms should be evaluated for colon cancer with either barium enema or colonoscopy. However, because many of the above symptoms may be difficult to identify on chart review, we do not recommend this as a quality indicator.

Staging and Preoperative Evaluation

Stage of disease is the most important determinant of prognosis in colorectal cancer. Multiple staging systems exist. The Dukes and the Modified Astler-Coller (MAC) classification schemes are most often used in treatment decisions, though the American Joint Committee on Cancer has also developed a staging system (Table 5.1). Bowel obstruction, bowel perforation, and adhesion or invasion of adjacent structures are indicators of poor prognosis (Steinberg et al., 1986), as are elevated pretreatment levels of carcinioembryonic antigen and CA 19-9. However, since these indications do not usually affect the initial choice of therapy, we do not recommend including them in a quality indicator (Filella et al., 1992).

Table 5.1

Definition of Stages of Colorectal Cancer

Stage	Dukes/ MAC	American Joint Committee on Cancer	Definitions of Stage for Quality Indicators
Stage 0		<u>Tis N0 M0</u> - carcinoma in situ	Carcinoma in situ
Stage I	Duke's A MAC A & B1	<u>T1 N0 M0</u> - tumor confined to bowel wall, invades submucosa <u>T2 N0 M0</u> - tumor confined to bowel wall, invades muscularis propria	Tumor is confined to bowel wall and does *not* invade all the way through the muscularis propria nor involve the subserosa or pericolic/perirectal tissues.
Stage II	Duke's B MAC B2 & B3	<u>T3 N0 M0</u> - tumor confined to bowel wall, invades through the muscularis propria into the subserosa <u>T4 N0 M0</u> - tumor perforates the visceral peritoneum or invades other organs or structures	Tumor is confined to bowel wall but invades all the way through the muscularis propria or involves the subserosa or pericolic/perirectal tissues.
Stage III	Duke's C MAC C1- C2	<u>Any T N1 M0</u> - metastases are present in 1-3 pericolic or perirectal lymph nodes <u>Any T N2 M0</u> - metastases are present in $\geq$ 4 pericolic or perirectal lymph nodes <u>Any T N3 M0</u> - metastases are present in any lymph node along the course of a named vascular trunk	Tumor involves lymph nodes.
Stage IV	Duke's D MAC D	<u>Any T Any N M1</u> - distant metastases are present	Distant metastases are present.

Since surgery is the mainstay of treatment of colorectal cancer, preoperative evaluation and staging should focus on obtaining information that would alter the planned operation or preclude surgery entirely (Vignati and Roberts 1993; Cohen, 1992). Since the incidence of synchronous carcinoma has been reported to be between two percent and 7.2 percent, all patients who undergo surgery should have a complete colonoscopy prior to the operation, to exclude a synchronous lesion that may necessitate a modification of the planned surgery (Vignati and Roberts 1993; Isler et al., 1987). If colonoscopy is unavailable, patients should be offered barium enema with sigmoidoscopy. Colonoscopy is preferred over barium enema because in a study of patients who had undergone both procedures, only half of the synchronous carcinomas found by colonoscopy were detected by barium enema (Isler et al., 1987). Our proposed indicator requires that all patients undergo colonoscopy or barium enema with sigmoidoscopy prior to surgical resection (Indicator 1).

For colon cancer, the value of routine preoperative imaging of the abdomen with either CT, MRI, or endocolic ultrasound, though often obtained, remains ill-defined. While there is consensus that patients with Stage I, II, and III colon cancer should undergo surgical resection with intent to cure, experts do not agree on the role of palliative surgical resection of the primary tumor in patients with Stage IV disease (CancerNet, 1997; Haskell and Berek, 1995). The extent of disease can be determined intraoperatively by palpation and ultrasound. The sensitivity of intraoperative ultrasound for detecting liver metastases is about 98 percent compared with 77 percent for CT scan (Parker et al., 1989). Therefore, if surgical resection is planned regardless of the stage of disease, preoperative imaging may not provide additional prognostic information. In addition, the accuracy of CT for predicting stage is poor, ranging from 48 percent to 64 percent (Balthazar et al., 1988; Freeny et al., 1986). Therefore, we do not recommend that routine preoperative imaging be included as a quality indicator.

For rectal cancer, the benefits of preoperative staging are clearer. In rectal cancer, preoperative evaluation centers on trying to determine if the tumor is limited (Stage I that may benefit from immediate local resection) or locally advanced (Stage II or III). The latter may benefit from preoperative radiation therapy to downstage the tumor and allow a sphincter-sparing operation, whereas a larger resection may have been required without it. Finally, if a patient already has metastatic disease (Stage IV), especially if the primary tumor is not causing symptoms, surgery may needlessly produce a loss of continence.

To guide initial treatment decisions, preoperative staging has an important role to play in rectal cancer. Clinical staging of rectal cancer includes a digital rectal exam with rigid proctoscopy. Using these techniques, a rectal tumor is considered to be at least a T3 lesion (making it at least Stage II cancer) if on digital rectal exam it is noted to be fixed in the pelvis. The accuracy of digital rectal exam in determining tumor penetration ranges from 48 percent to 85 percent, approaching the accuracy of pelvic CT (Beynon, 1986; Konishi et al., 1990; Milsom, 1990; Cohen et al., 1991; Glaser et al., 1990; Waizer et al., 1989). However, there is considerable inter-observer variation in the assessment of the stage of rectal carcinoma, and many lesions are not within reach of the examining finger (Nicholls et al., 1982). Unfortunately, digital rectal exam and proctoscopy do not allow for the assessment of lymph nodes (except for inguinal nodes which are not usually involved) or metastases.

Other techniques for the staging of rectal cancer include pelvic CT and MRI and endorectal ultrasound. While initial reports of pelvic CT in staging rectal cancer were extremely promising (Koehler et al., 1984; Theoni et al., 1981), inter-observer reliability has been reported to be only about 37 percent and test-retest reliability (reading of the same scan multiple times by the same radiologist) only 51 percent (Shank et al., 1990). In series comparing endorectal ultrasound with CT scan, endorectal ultrasound was better at detecting transmural penetration and lymph node spread, although CT was better at detecting liver metastases. In a comparative trial of MRI and CT, MRI did not compare favorably. The sensitivity of detecting lymph node metastases was 40 to 57 percent with CT and only 13 to 43 percent with MRI, with a specificity of 90 percent for both (Hodgman et al., 1986; Guinet et al., 1990).

Of the various imaging modalities, endorectal ultrasound has the best sensitivity and specificity at determining the extent of tumor penetration (67 to 97 percent and 50 to 92 percent, respectively) (Saitoh et al., 1986; Beynon et al., 1987; Konishi et al., 1990; Dershaw et al., 1990; Hildebrandt et al., 1990; Glaser et al., 1990; Beynon, 1989; Cohen et al., 1991; Di Candio et al., 1987; Milsom, 1990; Napolean et al., 1991; Dershaw et al., 1990). However, it is not as effective at evaluating lymph node metastases. Nonetheless, of the various imaging modalities, endorectal ultrasound probably has the greatest role in the preoperative staging of rectal cancer as it allows the surgeon to assess the degree of penetration, thus determining which tumors will be amenable to local excision, which will require wide excision, and which will benefit from preoperative radiation for downstaging in order to allow a sphincter saving operation. However, endorectal ultrasound is extremely operator dependent and is not yet widely available in the United States for the staging of rectal cancer (Hawes, 1993).

Given the complexity of the various clinical situations in rectal cancer that may or may not warrant preoperative imaging with endorectal ultrasound or CT scan, and the alternative surgical approaches that are largely at the discretion of the surgeon, we do not recommend a quality indicator for the routine use of any imaging studies in the preoperative evaluation of rectal cancer.

Other tests that are often obtained prior to surgery for colorectal cancer include liver function tests and the serum level of carcinoembryonic antigen (CEA)(Vignati and Roberts, 1993). However, the sensitivity and specificity of liver function tests do not make them useful for predicting metastatic disease in colorectal cancer. In one study of patients with elevated liver function tests prior to surgery for colorectal cancer, fewer than 50 percent had demonstrable metastatic disease at laparotomy, and, in long term follow-up they were no more likely to have metastases to the liver than patients without abnormal liver function tests (Tartter et al., 1984). Therefore, we do not recommend that routine screening of liver function tests be included in a quality indicator for the preoperative evaluation of colon cancer. CEA is a protein present in fetal tissue and in tumors of the gastrointestinal tract but not in normal adult intestinal tissue. Plasma concentrations of CEA may be elevated in colorectal tumors but they may also be normal, and CEA may also be elevated in non-malignant conditions such as in patients with chronic active hepatitis or in patients who smoke. Nonetheless, several large case series of patients with colorectal cancer have shown that an elevated preoperative CEA correlates with poorer survival, independent of stage of disease at diagnosis (Sener et al., 1989).

In practice, however, the level of the preoperative CEA does not change the initial management of patients with colorectal cancer. A preoperative CEA may be desirable if the clinician is going to be following the CEA postoperatively. However, since we are not recommending that serial CEA measurements be included in a quality indicator for follow-up (see discussion later), we do not recommend that they be included in a preoperative quality indicator either.

TREATMENT

Polyps

The quality indicators for the treatment of benign polyps are covered in Chapter 4. The incidence of carcinoma in situ in a polyp is approximately seven percent, while the incidence of invasive cancer in a polyp is approximately five percent (Stein and Coller, 1993). For a polyp that contains carcinoma in situ, curative treatment consists of complete excision of the polyp as there is no appreciable risk of spread (Stein and Coller, 1993). For polyps with invasive cancer, multiple case series have demonstrated that with favorable histologic conditions, the risk of developing recurrent or metastatic cancer is extremely low (approximately 2%) with complete polypectomy alone as treatment. Given that the operative mortality of a segmental colectomy is reported to be between 2.5 percent to 4.4 percent, the operative risks outweigh the potential benefits. However, in patients with unfavorable histologic features, the risk of cancer recurrence ranges from 15 percent (for invasion into the submucosa below the stalk or Level 4 invasion) to 48 percent (for a positive margin) (Stein and Coller, 1993). Other histologic features that predict cancer recurrence include lymphatic or venous invasion (45% risk) and Grade 3 differentiation (38% risk). Given the high risk of recurrent or metastatic disease from a polyp with unfavorable histologic features, experts recommend that these patients be offered a wide surgical resection (see sections on Localized Colon Cancer and Localized Rectal Cancer). Based upon this evidence, the American College of Gastroenterology recommends that only those polyps that are completely excised, not poorly differentiated, without vascular or lymphatic invasion, and with negative margins be treated with polypectomy alone; and for patients with polyps with poor prognostic features, the risk of surgical resection be weighed against the risk for death from metastatic cancer (Bond, 1993).

We recommend that the quality indicator for the treatment of malignant polyps specify that patients be offered a wide surgical resection if:

- the polyp is not completely excised,
- the margins are positive,
- lymphatic or venous invasion is present, or
- histology is Grade 3 or poorly differentiated (Indicator 2).

For patients who are treated with polypectomy alone (presumably those with favorable histologic features) the American College of Gastroenterology recommends a follow-up colonoscopy in three months to be sure that there is no abnormal residual tissue at the polypectomy site, followed by standard surveillance (Bond, 1993) (Indicator 3).

Localized Colon Cancer (Stage I, II, & III)

The standard treatment for colon cancer is surgery with wide resection and anastamosis (Nogueras and Jagelman, 1993). The aim of surgical treatment for cure is to remove the tumor and its lymphatic drainage and to provide adequate clear margins ensuring removal of the entire tumor burden. Wide surgical resection involves removing the entire tumor with a margin of bowel on either side along with the mesentery that contains the lymphatic drainage for that region of bowel. Retrospective studies have shown poorer survival rates with margins beyond the tumor of less than approximately 5 cm. However, since histopathologic studies have not identified intramural spread of tumor beyond 1.2 cm, most surgeons currently accept a 2 cm clear margin on either side of the tumor. Direct extension to surrounding organs does not preclude resection with curative intent as histopathologic examination of such "en bloc" resections confirms actual involvement only 48 to 84 percent of the time (Staniunas and Schoetz, 1993). Case series have shown a five year survival of 49 to 79 percent with en bloc resection compared with zero to 17 percent without (McGlone et al., 1982; Gall, 1987).

Approximately 25 percent of patients have distant metastases and are not candidates for surgical resection with curative intent. Several case series have suggested a benefit in survival and symptoms from a surgical resection with palliative intent; however, experts disagree on the merits of this approach (O'Connell, 1997). For this reason, we will limit our quality indicator for the surgical treatment of colon cancer to those cases where the intent is cure (Stages I to III). Wide surgical resection should be offered to all patients with Stages I to III colon cancer, including those with locally invasive disease, unless coexisting medical problems substantially increase the mortality risk of the surgical procedure itself. In order to operationalize this as an indicator, evidence of wide resection will be obtained from the pathology report as follows: The surgical specimen must include the tumor with at least 2 cm of bowel on either side, and there must be lymph nodes present. Age alone is not a contraindication to aggressive treatment for colorectal cancer as acceptable mortality and morbidity are achieved even in patients over age 70 (Fitzgerald, 1993) (Indicator 4). As an assessment of the technical quality of the surgical resection, for patients with Stage I colon cancer or Stage II and III colon cancer that does not invade other organs, the surgical specimen should have negative margins (Indicator 5).

Adjuvant Therapy of Colon Cancer

Randomized trials have shown a benefit for adjuvant chemotherapy in Stage III colon cancer (The Medical Letter, 1996; Moertel, 1994). Results of two randomized controlled trials that demonstrated approximately a 30 percent reduction in the overall mortality for patients with Stage III colon cancer treated with 5-FU and levamisole (Moertel et al., 1990; Laurie et al., 1989; Moertel, 1995). Based on these results, an NIH Consensus Conference convened in 1990 recommended that all patients with Stage III colon cancer be offered adjuvant chemotherapy for one year (5-FU with levamisole) within six weeks of their surgical resection (NIH Consensus Statement Online, 1990). In addition, the combination of 5-FU with leucovorin has been shown to have a similar benefit on overall and disease-free survival in several randomized trials when compared with a 5-FU, semustine, and vincristine regimen, and when compared with no adjuvant treatment (Wolmark et al., 1993; IMPA of Colon Cancer Trials 1995; O'Connell, 1997). Maturing data from trials comparing various dosage schedules of 5-FU and leucovorin with the now standard 5-FU and levamisole did not demonstrate a significant difference between them (Haller et al., 1996; Wolmark, 1996).

For Stage II colon cancer, there was a non-significant trend toward improved disease-free and overall survival in one of the trials of adjuvant 5-FU and leucovorin (Moertel, 1990). Similarly, analysis of pooled data from several National Surgical Adjuvant Breast and Bowel Project (NSABP) trials suggested a survival advantage comparable to that seen in Stage III patients with adjuvant chemotherapy (Mamounas et al., 1996). None of the studies to date have demonstrated a clear benefit for adjuvant chemotherapy in Stage II patients (Laurie et al., 1989; International Multicentre Pooled Analysis of Colon Cancer Trials, 1995). In keeping with these data, the NIH Consensus Conference in 1990 did not make a recommendation regarding adjuvant chemotherapy in Stage II colon cancer (NIH Consensus Statement Online, 1990).

Patients with Stage III colon cancer should be offered adjuvant chemotherapy with one of the following published 5-FU-containing regimens, beginning 21 days to six weeks after surgery (The Medical Letter, 1996) (Indicator 6):

1. 5-FU 450 mg/m^2 rapid intravenous injection daily for five consecutive days followed by weekly 5-FU treatments, at the same dose, beginning 28 days from the start of treatment and continuing for 48 weeks, and levamisole 50 mg orally every eight hours for three days beginning with the first dose of 5-FU and repeated every two weeks for 52 weeks.

2. Leucovorin 200 mg/m^2 followed by 5-FU 370-400 mg/m^2 rapid intravenous injection daily for five consecutive days repeated every 28 days for at least six cycles and not more than 12 cycles (International Multicentre Pooled Analysis of Colon Cancer Trials 1995, Haller et al., 1996; Wolmark et al., 1996)

3. Leucovorin 20 mg/m^2 followed by 5-FU 370-425 mg/m^2 rapid intravenous injection daily for five consecutive days repeated every 28 days for at least six cycles and not more than 12 cycles.

4. Leucovorin 500 mg/m^2 followed by 5-FU 500 mg/m^2 intravenous infusion weekly, for six weeks of an eight week cycle, for at least six cycles and not more than 12 cycles.

Localized Rectal Cancer

Like colon cancer, the mainstay of treatment for rectal cancer is wide surgical resection of the primary and regional lymph nodes with anastamosis, provided there is sufficient distal rectum to allow for it. Surgery can be accomplished either by the sphincter-sparing low anterior resection (usually necessitates tumor at least 7 to 8 cm of the anal verge) or the sphincter-sacrificing abdominal perineal resection for lesions too distal to permit low anterior resection. Overall survival is comparable with the two approaches, though a greater number of local recurrences occur with the abdominal perineal resection (18-21% versus 7% for low anterior resection) (Butcher, 1971; Malt, 1974; Slanetz, 1972; Mayo, 1960; Mayo, 1958; Balsley, 1973).

Stage I rectal cancer has a high cure rate with surgery alone, with 90 to 95 percent disease-free survival at five years (Heald et al., 1986). While the standard surgical procedure would be a low anterior resection or abdominal perineal resection as described in the proceeding paragraph, retrospective series suggest that patients with small (< 4 cm) well- to moderately-well differentiated adenocarcinoma with no lymphatic or venous invasion treated with full-thickness local excision that results in negative margins have comparable outcomes in selected populations, with or without radiation therapy (Minsky, 1995; Buess, 1995; Scholefield et al., 1995; Heimann, 1992; Bailey et al., 1992; Willett et al., 1994). Other treatments including endocavitary irradiation and electrofulguration have been described; however, these have not been compared in randomized trials to surgery (CancerNet PDQ, 1997). Our proposed quality indicators for Stage I rectal cancer require that patients be offered definitive surgical treatment with low anterior resection or abdominal perineal resection, or have a full-thickness local excision described in the pathology report to have "negative margins" (Indicators 7 and 9).

Patients with Stage II and III rectal cancer are at high risk for local and systemic recurrences. While only five to ten percent of patients with Stage I disease will recur, 25 to 30 percent of those with Stage II will relapse. Up to 50 percent of patients with Stage III rectal cancer will recur (Heald et al., 1986). It is believed that the principal reason for patients with rectal cancer having a higher local recurrence rate than patients with colon cancer is the difficulty in obtaining clear radial margins given the constraints of the pelvic anatomy. Randomized trials of preoperative or postoperative radiation therapy alone have demonstrated a significant decrease in local recurrence rates without any impact on overall survival (Gerard, 1988; Thomas, 1988; Fisher et al., 1988; Mohiuddin et al., 1991). However, several studies have demonstrated an increase in both disease-free survival and overall survival for patients with Stage II and III rectal cancer when chemotherapy is combined with radiation therapy in the postoperative period (Thomas, 1988; The Medical Letter, 1996; Pahlman, 1995; Freedman et al., 1995; Krook et al., 1991; Gastrointestinal Tumor Study Group, 1992; Moertel, 1994).

This lead the NIH Consensus Conference on colorectal cancer in 1990 to conclude that all patients with Stage II or III rectal cancer should be offered perioperative combined modality therapy with chemotherapy and high-dose pelvic radiation therapy (4500 to 5500 cGy). While the initial studies of combined modality therapy used 5-FU and semustine, subsequent randomized trials have found that 5-FU alone is equally effective (and semustine has been shown to be leukemogenic)(Gastrointestinal Tumor Study Group 1984 and 1992). Though one study did demonstrate a modest survival with prolonged 5-FU infusion over bolus infusion of 5-FU during radiation therapy, either protocol with or without the addition of leucovorin is considered standard (O'Conell et al., 1994). For patients with low rectal tumors, one study has shown that high-dose preoperative radiation therapy may allow preservation of anal sphincter function (and continence) upon resection of the tumor (Mohiuddin et al., 1991). Our recommended quality indicators for the treatment of Stage II and III rectal cancer state that patients should be offered complete surgical resection with either a low anterior resection or abdominal perineal resection (Indicator 8), followed by postoperative 5-FU and radiation therapy of 4500 to 5500 cGy to the pelvis, or preoperative radiation therapy, with or without 5-FU chemotherapy, followed by complete surgical resection (Indicator 10).

Isolated Liver Metastases (Stage IV)

For patients who have isolated liver metastases, either at the time of initial diagnosis or who later develop them as the only site of recurrence, surgical resection, if it is technically feasible, offers a hope of cure and in multiple case series has a five year survival of approximately 25 percent (Fong, 1995; Taylor, 1996; Steele et al., 1991; Pedersen et al., 1994; Coppa et al., 1985; Adson et al., 1984; Scheele et al., 1990; Gayowski et al., 1994; Scheele et al., 1991). The number of historical controls that have lived beyond five years are strikingly few. Randomized trials have not been performed because the investigators have not believed them to be ethical. The operative mortality has been reported between three and seven percent (Fong, 1995; Taylor, 1996). Factors that predict a more favorable course after liver resection of colorectal metastases include tumor size less than 4 cm, fewer than four metastases, unilobar involvement, and original stage of disease (Gayowski et al., 1994; Scheele et al., 1991). This evidence suggests that selected patients will benefit from resection of colorectal metastases to the liver. From chart review alone, however, it would prove difficult to identify those patients who would possibly have benefitted. In addition, only five percent of patients with colorectal cancer develop isolated liver metastases that appear amenable to surgical resection (Scheele et al., 1990). Therefore, given the small numbers of patients affected, and the difficulty in identifying those patients who would benefit, we have not included resection of isolated liver metastases as a quality indicator.

Hepatic artery infusion of chemotherapy is another treatment occasionally used in the treatment of colorectal liver metastases. Studies have shown that while this approach achieves a higher response rate, there is no improvement in overall survival (Kemeny et al., 1987; Chang, 1987; Wagman, Rougier et al., 1992; Kemeny et al., 1993; Meta-analysis Group in Cancer, 1996).

Metastatic Colorectal Cancer (Stage IV)

Approximately 50 percent of patients have metastatic disease on presentation. Unfortunately, there is no therapy for metastatic colon cancer that has been shown to improve survival. Chemotherapy has been used for palliation of symptoms with the hope of prolonging survival (The Medical Letter, 1996; Moertel, 1994; Kemeny et al., 1993). 5-FU based regimens are the standard, and multiple trials have been conducted comparing 5-FU alone with 5-FU modulated by varying agents including methotrexate, leucovorin, and interferon alpha, all in varying dosage schedules. While generally the modulation of 5-FU with these agents improved the response rate (number of cases where the tumor size decreases during the course of treatment), there has not been a consistent improvement in overall survival demonstrated with any of these protocols, and treatment-related toxicities have generally been worse with the combination and higher dosage regimens (Erlichman et al., 1988; Doroshow et al., 1990; Petrelli et al., 1989; Petrelli et al., 1987; Leichman et al., 1995; Buroker et al., 1994; Poon et al., 1989; Advanced Colorectal Cancer Meta-analysis Project, 1994; Hill et al., 1995; Corfu-A Study Group, 1995). Likewise, continuous infusion of 5-FU via an ambulatory infusion pump has been associated with a modest increase in the response rate but no improvement in overall survival (Lokich et al., 1989; Leichman, 1995). Irinotecan is a new drug that was approved by the FDA in June of 1996, under

89

the provisions of the accelerated approval process, for use in metastatic colorectal cancer that has recurred or progressed on standard chemotherapy (Micromedex Healthcare Series Drug Information DRUGDEX(R) System 1975-1997). In phase II studies, irinotecan had a response rate of 23 percent to 32 percent in metastatic colorectal cancer. However, no randomized studies of its efficacy have been performed, and no data are available on its effect on disease-free or overall survival (Rothenberg, 1996; Conti, 1996). Surprisingly, given that the goal of therapy in metastatic disease is palliation, few studies have included performance status, symptoms, or quality of life as endpoints (Buroker et al., 1994; Poon, 1989; Sullivan, 1995; Laufman et al., 1993). One study comparing 5-FU modulated by high versus low dose leucovorin found no difference in quality of life outcomes. Another study included six arms of 5-FU modulated by varying doses of leucovorin, methotrexate, or cisplatin. The low dose leucovorin arm demonstrated a higher response rate for improvement in performance status, weight gain, and palliation of symptoms (Buroker et al., 1994; Poon et al., 1989). This regimen also had the lowest drug cost (Poon, 1989).

Palliative surgery also has a role in metastatic colorectal cancer, especially to relieve obstruction or treat bleeding or perforation. In addition, several case series have suggested a benefit in survival and symptoms from a surgical resection with palliative intent. However, experts disagree on the merits of this approach (CancerNet PDQ, 1997; Haskell, 1995).

Given the variety of clinical scenarios, the absence of strong evidence that any treatment improves survival or quality of life in all or even most patients, and the lack of expert consensus, we do not recommend a quality indicator for the treatment of metastatic colorectal cancer.

Toxicity

Most chemotherapy regimens for colorectal cancer, whether adjuvant or palliative, include 5-FU, and the main toxicities of those regimens are secondary to the 5-FU. 5-FU toxicity varies with the dose and the schedule (daily, weekly, continuous infusion), but may include nausea, vomiting, diarrhea, leukopenia, stomatitis, and erythrodysesthesia (hand foot syndrome) (The Medical Letter, 1996). The dose limiting toxicity (Grade 3 or 4) for the five-daily fast intravenous infusion is generally neutropenia (3 to 47 percent of patients) or stomatitis (3 to 28 percent), and for the weekly intravenous infusion, diarrhea (13 to 40 percent). These effects require that chemotherapy be witheld until symptoms resolve and often result in dose reduction as well (The Medical Letter, 1996; Erlichman et al., 1988; Doroshow et al., 1990; Petrelli et al., 1989; Petrelli et al., 1987; Leichman et al., 1995; Poon et al., 1989; Moertel et al., 1990; Laurie et al., 1989; Wolmark et al., 1993; International Multicentre Pooled Analysis of Colon Cancer Trials, 1995). The fatal complications of therapy with 5-FU are usually related to sepsis with neutropenia or severe diarrhea. We recommend two quality indicators for all patients receiving chemotherapy with 5-FU. The first requires that all patients have a CBC not more that 48 hours prior to the first day of 5-FU in each cycle of chemotherapy (Indicator 11). The second states that patients with Grade 3 or 4 toxicity (a WBC less than 2,000, stomatitis that prevents eating, or diarrhea of seven or more stools a day) should have chemotherapy witheld until the symptoms resolve (Indicator 12).

Recurrent Colon Cancer

One third of patients diagnosed with colorectal cancer will develop recurrent disease (Asbun, 1993; Safi, 1993). Most will have distant metastases, but 21 percent will have an isolated local recurrence. Local recurrence is more common in rectal cancer, comprising approximately 50 percent of recurrences. An additional 25 percent have isolated hepatic metastases, and approximately four percent present with isolated pulmonary lesions. Local recurrences may present at the site of the anastamosis or more commonly in the bed of the primary carcinoma. Surgery is the only hope for cure in these patients. Case series of selected patients who have undergone a second resection report median lengths of survival after resection of 35 to 85 months (Michelassi et al., 1990). The approach to isolated liver metastases is discussed above. For the rare case of an isolated pulmonary metastasis, wedge excision is an option with curative potential. In a series of 139 patients with solitary pulmonary metastases who underwent resection, the five year survival rate was 30.5 percent and the 20 year-survival rate was 16.2 percent (McAfee, 1992). Again, given the variety of clinical scenarios for a relatively few number of patients, we believe it would be difficult to

91

implement a quality indicator for recurrent colorectal cancer and do not recommend one.

FOLLOW-UP AND POSTOPERATIVE SURVEILLANCE

Of patients who undergo a surgical resection with curative intent, 30 percent to 50 percent will develop recurrent disease (Vignati et al., 1993; Safi et al., 1993). The goal of postoperative surveillance after curative resection for colorectal carcinoma is the detection of recurrent tumor at a stage when it is still curable and the prevention or early detection of a metachronous carcinoma. However, to date there have been no large-scale randomized trials to document the efficacy of a postoperative monitoring program and intensive surveillance of colorectal cancer patients after resection with curative intent remains controversial (Steele, 1993; Safi, 1993; Moertel et al., 1993).

As there is no literature on the efficacy of surveillance of patients with metastatic colorectal cancer, we recommend that the quality indicator be limited to patients with potentially curable disease (Stages I to III). Methods of surveillance commonly used to follow patients with colorectal cancer who have undergone a curative resection include periodic history and physical examination, serial CEA measurements, periodic imaging studies, and colonoscopy (Vignati et al., 1993).

In two studies, positive findings on a thorough history and physical exam provided the first indication of recurrent disease in up to 48 percent of patients (Beart et al., 1983; Deveney et al., 1984). As periodic history and physical examination can be accomplished without special technology and is relatively inexpensive we will include it in our quality indicator for the follow-up of Stages I to III colorectal cancer. Since 85 percent of colorectal cancers recur in the first three years, our proposed quality indicator for follow-up requires a history and physical exam by a physician at least every six months for three years after initiation of treatment (Indicator 13) (Vignati et al., 1993).

Serial measurement of serum CEA levels has been widely accepted as a way to identify recurrences while they may still be resectable for cure. In one analysis of 146 asymptomatic patients who underwent a second look operation only because of a rise in CEA, 95 percent had recurrences and, of these, 58 percent were resectable for potential cure. Of those patients who were reoperated upon, the five year survival rate was approximately 30 percent (Martin et al., 1985). However, other large retrospective studies found a year disease-free survival rate after salvage surgery of two percent in CEA-monitored patients; the one year disease free survival of patients who underwent salvage surgery with no CEA monitoring was identical (Moertel et al., 1995; Minton et al., 1985). No randomized prospective trials have been performed to evaluate the efficacy of CEA in the postoperative surveillance of colorectal cancer. While many physicians may choose to follow CEA levels in their patients with colorectal cancer, given the absence of clear data in the literature, we will not include CEA monitoring in our quality indicators for the follow-up of colorectal cancer.

Periodic imaging studies, including CT or MRI of the abdomen, chest x-ray or CT of the chest, and endorectal ultrasound are all used to detect recurrent colorectal cancer. Unfortunately, there are no controlled studies to provide information on the efficacy of these studies in monitoring patients with colorectal cancer (Vignati et al., 1993; Kagan et al., 1991). We will therefore not include any imaging studies in our quality indicators for the follow-up of colorectal cancer.

There are no controlled studies of postoperative surveillance for colorectal cancer with colonoscopy. Recent consensus guidelines, developed by the American Gastroenterological Association (AGA) and endorsed by the American Cancer Society and the American Society of Colon and Rectal Surgeons recommend a colonoscopy or double contrast barium enema (DCBE) within a year of curative surgery if it did not occur preoperatively (Indicator 14). If the colonoscopy or DCBE is normal at three years post-surgery, the test should then be performed every five years (Indicator 15) (Winawer et al., 1997). This indicator is similar to the AGA recommendations for adenomatous polyps, which are based upon randomized controlled trials in that population. A retrospective study of 290 patients who underwent resection with curative intent for colorectal cancer and were followed with colonoscopy (initially every six months, and every one to two years after the first year) suggests that there might be a benefit for routine postoperative surveillance with colonoscopy (Winawer et al., 1997). These authors found that 75 percent of patients who had asymptomatic recurrences identified by colonoscopy were able to undergo a second resection compared with only 16 percent of patients whose recurrences were identified when they presented with symptoms (Lautenbach et al., 1994). Several other case series have found that up to ten percent of patients may have metachronous cancers discovered by screening colonoscopy, although, a much smaller percentage were actually asymptomatic at the time (Barlow et al., 1993; Patchett et al., 1993). Even though conclusive data regarding the efficacy of postoperative surveillance for colorectal cancer with either colonoscopy or double contrast barium enema are lacking, given the current evidence in its favor and its widespread acceptance as the standard of care, we will include it in the quality indicator for follow-up of patients with Stage I to III colorectal cancer (Indicator 15).

REFERENCES

Adson MA, van Heerden JA, Adson MH, et al. 1984. Resection of hepatic metastases from colorectal cancer. *Archives of Surgery* 119: 647-651.

Advanced Colorectal Cancer Meta-analysis Project. 1994. Meta-analysis of randomized trials testing the biochemical modulation of fluorouracil by methotrexate in metastatic colorectal cancer. *Journal of Clinical Oncology* 12: 960-969.

Asbun HJ, and Hughes KS. 1993. Management of recurrent and metastatic colorectal carcinoma. *Surgical Clinics of North America* 73: 145-166.

Bailey HR, Huval WV, Max E, et al. 1992. Local excision of carcinoma of the rectum for cure. *Surgery* 2: 555-561.

Balsley I, Fenger HJ, Jensen H-E, Kragelund E, and Nielsen J. 1973. Carcinoma of the rectum: treatment by anterior resection or abdominoperineal excision? *Diseases of the Colon and Rectum* 16: 206-210.

Balthazar EJ, Megibow AJ, Hulnick D, et al. 1988. Carcinoma of the colon: Detection and preoperative staging by CT. *American Journal of Radiology* 150: 301-306.

Barlow AP, and Thompson MH. 1993. Colonoscopic follow-up after resection for colorectal cancer: a selective policy. *British Journal of Surgery* 80: 781-784.

Beart RW Jr, and O'Connell MJ. 1983. Postoperative follow-up of patients with carcinoma of the colon. *Mayo Clinic Proceedings* 58: 361-363.

Beynon J. 1989. An evaluation of the role of rectal endosonography in rectal cancer. *Annals of the Royal College of Surgeons of England* 71: 131-139.

Beynon JMcC, Mortensen NJ, Foy DMA, Channer JL, Virjee J, and Goddard P. 1986. Pre-operative assessment of local invasion in rectal cancer: digital examination, endoluminal sonography or computed tomography? *British Journal of Surgery* 73: 1015-7.

Beynon J, Mortensen NJM, Channer JL, et al. 1989. Preoperative assessment of mesorectal lymph node involvement in rectal cancer. *British Journal of Surgery* 76: 276-279.

Beynon J, Roe AM, Foy DM, Channer JL, Virjee J, and Mortensen NJ. 1987. Preoperative staging of local invasion in rectal cancer using intraluminal ultrasound. *Journal of the Royal Society of Medicine* 80: 23-6.

Bond JH, and for the Practice Parameters Committee of the American College of Gastroenterology. 1993. Position paper. Polyp guideline: diagnosis, treatment, and surveillance for patients with nonfamilial colorectal polyps. *Archives of Internal Medicine* 19: 836-843.

Buess BF. 1995. Local surgical treatment of rectal cancer. *European Journal of Cancer* 31A: 1233-37.

Buroker TR, O'Connell MJ, Wienand S, Krook JE, Gerstner JB, et al. 1994. Randomized comparison of two schedules of fluorouracil and leucovorin in the treatment of advanced colorectal cancer. *Journal of Clinical Oncology* 12: 14-20.

Butcher HR Jr. 1971. Carcinoma of the rectum. Choice between anterior resetcion and abdominal perineal resection of the rectum. *Cancer* 28: 204-207.

CancerNet PDQ Information for Health Care Professionals. March 1997. *Rectal Cancer*. National Cancer Institute.

CancerNet PDQ Information for Health Care Professionals. March 1997. *Colon Cancer*. National Cancer Institute.

Chang AE, Schneider PD, Sugarbaker PH, Simpson C, Culnane M, and Steinberg SM. 1987. A prospective randomized trial of regional versus systemic continuous 5-fluorodeoxyuridine chemotherapy in the treatment of colorectal liver metastases. *Annals of Surgery* 206: 685-693.

Cohen AM. 1992. Preoperative evaluation of patients with primary colorectal cancer. *Cancer* 7: 1328-1332.

Cohen JL, Grotz RL, Welch JP, et al. 1991. Intrarectal sonography. A new technique for the assessment of rectal tumors. *American Surgeon* 57: 459-462.

Conti JA, Kemeny NE, Saltz LB, Huang Y, Tong WP, Chou TC, et al. 1996. Irinotecan is an active agent in untreated patients with metastatic colorectal cancer. *Journal of Clinical Oncology* 14: 709-715.

Coppa GF, Eng K, Ranson JH, Gouge TH, and Localio SA. 1985. Hepatic resection for metastatic colon and rectal cancer. An evaluation of preoperative and postoperative factors. *Annals of Surgery* 202: 203-208.

Corfu-A Study Group. 1995. Phase III randomized study of two fluorouracil combination with either interferon alfa-2a or leucovorin for advanced colorectal cancer. *Journal of Clinical Oncology* 13: 921-928.

Dershaw DD, Warren EE, Cohen AM, and Sigurdson ER. 1990. Transrectal ultrasonography of rectal carcinoma. *Cancer* 66: 2336-40.

Deveney KE, and Way LW. 1984. Follow-up of patients with colorectal cancer. *American Journal of Surgery* 148: 717-722.

Di Candio G, Mosca F, Compatelli A, et al. 1987. Endosonographic staging of rectal carcinoma. *Gastrointestinal Radiology* 12: 289-295.

Doroshow JH, Multhauf P, Leong L, Margolin K, Litchfield T, Akman S, et al. 1990. Prospective randomized comparison of fluorouracil versus fluorouracil and high-dose continuous infusion leucovorin calcium for the treatment of advanced measurable colorectal cancer in patients previously unexposed to chemotherapy. *Journal of Clinical Oncology* 8: 491-501.

Erlichman C, Fine S, Wong A, and Elhakim T. 1988. A randomized trial of fluorouracil and folinic acid in patients with metastatic colorectal carcinoma. *Journal of Clinical Oncology* 6: 469-475.

Filella X, Molina R, Grau JJ, et al. 1992. Prognostic value of CA 19-9 levels in colorectal cancer. *Annals of Surgery* 216: 55-59.

Fisher B, Wolmark N, Rockette H, et al. 1988. Postoperative adjuvant chemotherapy or radiation therapy for rectal cancer: results from the NSABP protocol R-01. *Journal of the National Cancer Institute* 80: 21-29.

Fitzgerald SD, Longo WE, Daniel GL, et al. 1993. Advanced colorectal neoplasia in the high-risk elderly patient: is surgical resection justified? *Diseases of the Colon and Rectum* 36: 161-166.

Fong Y, Blumgart LH, and Cohen A. 1995. Surgical treatment of colorectal metastases to the liver. *CA Cancer a Journal for Clinicians* 45: 50-62.

Freedman GM, and Coia LR. 1995. Adjuvant and neoadjuvant treatment of rectal cancer. *Seminars in Oncology* 22: 611-24.

Freeny PC, Marks WM, Ryan JA, et al. 1986. Colorectal Carcinoma evaluation with CT: Preoperative staging and detection of postoperative recurrence. *Radiology* 158: 347-353.

Gall FP, Tonak J, and Altendorf A. 1987. Multivisceral resections in colorectal cancer. *Diseases of the Colon and Rectum* 30: 337-341.

Gastrointestinal Tumor Study Group. 1984. Adjuvant therapy of colon cancer. Results of a prospectively randomized trial. *New England Journal of Medicine* 310: 737-743.

Gastrointestinal Tumor Study Group. 1992. Radiation therapy and fluorouracil with or without semustine for the treatment of patients with surgical adjuvant adenocarcinoma of the rectum. *Journal of Clinical Oncology* 10: 549-557.

Gayowski TJ, Shunzaburo I, Madariaga JR, Selby R, Todo S, et al. 1994. Experience in hepatic resection for metastatic colorectal cancer: analysis of clinical and pathological risk factors. *Surgery* 116: 703-711.

Gerard A, Buyse M, Mordlinger B, et al. 1988. Preoperative radiotherapy as adjuvant treatment in rectal cancer: final results of a randomized study of the European Organization for Research and Treatment of Cancer (EORTC). *Annals of Surgery* 208: 606-614.

Glaser F, Schlag P, and Herfarth C. 1990. Endorectal ultrasonography for the assessment of invasion of rectal tumours and lymph node involvement. *British Journal of Surgery* 77: 883-7.

Guinet C, Buy JN, Ghossian MA, Sezeur A, Mallet A, Bigot JM, et al. 1990. Comparison of magnetic resonance imaging and computed tomography in the preoperative staging of rectal cancer. *Archives of Surgery* 125: 383-8.

Haller DG, Catalano PJ, Macdonald JS, Mayer RJ, for ECOG, SWOG, and and CALGB. 1996. Flurouracil (FU), leucovorin (LV) and levamisole (LEV) adjuvant therapy for colon cancer: preliminary results of INT-0089. *Proceedings of ASCO* 15 (486): 211.

Haskell CM, and Berek JS, Eds. 1995. *Cancer Treatment*, 4th edition ed.Philadelphia, Pennsylvania: W.B. Saunders Company.

Hawes RH. 1993. New Staging Techniques. Endoscopic ultrasound. *Cancer* 71 (Suppl 12): 4207-4213.

Heald RJ, and Ryall RD. 1986. Recurrence and survival after total mesorectal excision for rectal cancer. *Lancet* 1 (8496): 1479-1482.

Heimann TM, Oh C, Steinhagen RM, Greenstein AJ, Perez C, and Aufses AH Jr. 1992. Surgical treatment of tumors of the distal rectum with sphincter preservation. *Annals of Surgery* 216: 432-6.

Hildebrandt U, Klein T, Feifel G, et al. 1990. Endosonography of pararectal lymph nodes. *Diseases of the Colon and Rectum* 33: 863-868.

Hill M, Norman A, Cunningham D, Findlay M, Nicolson V, Hill A, et al. 1995. Royal Marsden phase III trial of fluorouracil with or without interferon alfa-2b in advanced colorectal cancer. *Journal of Clinical Oncology* 13: 1297-1302.

Hodgman CG, MacCarty RL, Wolff BG, May GR, Berquist TH, Sheedy PF II, et al. 1986. Preoperative staging of rectal carcinoma by computed tomography and 0.15 T magnetic resonance imaging: preliminary report. *Diseases of the Colon and Rectum* 29: 446-50.

International Multicentre Pooled Analysis of Colon Cancer Trials. 1995. Efficacy of adjuvant fluorouracil and folinic acid in colon cancer. *Lancet* 345: 939-944.

Isler JJ, Brown PC, and Lewis FG. 1987. The role of preoperative colonoscopy in colorectal cancer. *Diseases of the Colon and Rectum* 30: 435-439.

Kagan AR, and Steckel RJ. 1991. Routine imaging studies for the posttreatment surveillance of breast and colorectal carcinoma. *Journal of Clinical Oncology* 9: 837-842.

Kemeny N, Cohen A, Seiter K, Conti JA, Sigurdson ER, Tao Y, Niedzwiecki D, Botet J, and Budd A. 1993. Randomized trial of hepatic arterial floxuridine, mitomycin, and carmustine versus floxuridine alone in previously treated patients with liver metastases from colorectal cancer. *Journal of Clinical Oncology* 11: 330-335.

Kemeny N, Daly J, Reichman B, Geller N, Botet J, and Oderman P. 1987. Intrahepatic or systemic infusion of fluorodeoxyuridine in patients with liver metastases from colorectal carcinoma. A randomized trial. *Archives of Internal Medicine* 107: 459-465.

Kemeny N, Lokich JJ, Anderson N, and Ahlgren JD. 1993. Recent advances in the treatment of advanced colorectal cancer. *Cancer* 71: 9-18.

Koehler PR, Feldberg MAM, and van Waes PFGM. 1984. Preoperative staging of rectal cancer with computerized tomography: accuracy, efficacy, and effect on patient management. *Cancer* 512-6.

Konishi G, Ugajin H, Ito K, and Kanazawa K. 1990. Endorectal ultrasonography with a 7.5 Mhz linear array scanner for the assessment of invasion of rectal carcinoma. *International Journal of Colorectal Disease* 5: 15-20.

Krook JE, Moertel CG, Gunderson LL, et al. 1991. Effective surgical adjuvant therapy for high-risk rectal carcinoma. *New England Journal of Medicine* 324: 709-715.

Laufman LR, Bukowski RM, Collier MA, Sullivan BA, McKinnis RA, Clendennin NJ, Guaspari A, and Brenckman WD. 1993. A randomized, double-blind trial of fluorouracil plus placebo versus fluorouracil plus oral leucovorin in patients with metastatic colorectal cancer. *Journal of Clinical Oncology* 11: 1888-1893.

Laurie JA, Moertel CG, Fleming TR, Wieand HS, Leigh JE, Rubin J, et al. 1989. Surgical adjuvant therapy of large-vowel carcinoma: an evaluation of levamisole and the combination of levamisole and fluorouracil. *Journal of Clinical Oncology* 7: 1447-1456.

Lautenbach E, Forde KA, and Neugut AI. 1994. Benefits of colonoscopic surveillance after curative resection of colorectal cancer. *Annals of Surgery* 220: 206-211.

Leichman CG, Fleming TR, Muggia FM, Tangen CM, et al. 1995. Phase II study of fluorouracil and its modulation in advanced colorectal cancer: a Southwest Oncology Group Study. *Journal of Clinical Oncology* 13: 1303-1311.

Levitan N. 1993. Chemotherapy in colorectal cancer. *Surgical Clinics of North America* 73: 183-198.

Lokich JJ, Ahlgren JD, Gullow JJ, Philips JA, and Fryer JG. 1989. A prospective randomized comparison of continuous infusion fluorouracil with a conventional bolus schedule in metastatic colorectal carcinoma: a Mid-Atlantic Oncology Program study. *Journal of Clinical Oncology* 7: 425-432.

Malt RA, and Nundy S. 1974. Rectal carcinoma. Abdominoperineal and anterior resections. *Surgical Clinics of North America* 54: 741-750.

Mamounas EP, Rockette H, Jones J, Wieand S, et al. 1996. Comparative efficacy of adjuvant chemotherapy in patients with Dukes' B vs Dukes' C colon cancer: results from four NSABP adjuvant studies (C-01, C-02, C-03, C-04). *Proceedings of ASCO* 15 (461): 205.

Martin EW, Minton JP, and Carey LC. 1985. CEA directed second-look surgery in the asymptomatic patient after primary resection of colorectal carcinoma. *Annals of Surgery* 202: 310-317.

Mayo C, and Cullen PK. July 1960. An evaluation of the one stage low anterior resection. *Surgery, Gynecology, Obstetrics* 2: 82-86.

Mayo C, Laberge MY, and Hardy WM. June 1958. Five year survival after anterior resection for carcinoma of the rectum and rectosigmoid. *Surgery, Gynecology, Obstetrics* 109: 695-698.

McAfee MK, Allen MS, Trasted VF, Ilstrup DM, Deschamps C, and Pairolero PC. 1992. Colorectal lung metastases: result of surgical excision. *Annals of Thoracic Surgery* 53: 780-6.

McGlone TP, Bernie WA, and Elliott DW. 1982. Survival following extended operation for extracolonic invasion by colon cancer. *Archives of Surgery* 117: 595-599.

Meta-analysis Group in Cancer. 1996. Reappraisal of hepatic arterial infusion in the treatment of nonresectable liver metastases from colorectal cancer. *Journal of the National Cancer Institute* 88: 252-8.

Michelassi F, Vannucci L, Ayala JJ, et al. 1990. Local recurrence after curative resection of colorectal adenocarcinoma. *Surgery* 108: 787-793.

Micromedex Healthcare Series Drug Information. 1997. DRUGDEX(R) System. *Drug Evaluation Monographs* 91.

Milsom JW, and Graffner H. 1990. Intrarectal ultrasonography in rectal cancer staging and in the evaluation of pelvic disease. Clinical uses of intrarectal ultrasound. *Annals of Surgery* 212: 602-606.

Minsky BD. 1995. Conservative treatment of rectal cancer with local excision and postoperative radiation therapy. *European Journal of Cancer* 31A: 1343-6.

Minton JP, Hoehn JL, Gerber DM, et al. 1985. Results of a 400 patient carcinoembryonic antigen second-look colorectal cancer study. *Cancer* 55: 1284-1290.

Moertel CG. 1994. Chemotherapy for colorectal cancer. *New England Journal of Medicine* 330: 1136-1142.

Moertel CG, Fleming TR, Macdonald JS, et al. 1993. An evaluation of the carcinoembryonic antigen (CEA) test for monitoring patients with resected colon cancer. *Journal of the American Medical Association* 270: 943-947.

Moertel CG, Fleming TR, Macdonal JS, Haller DG, et al. 1995. Fluorouracil plus levamisole as effective adjuvant therapy after resection of Stage III colon carcinoma: a final report. *Archives of Internal Medicine* 122: 321-326.

Moertel CG, Fleming TR, MacDonald JS, Haller DG, Laurie JA, et al. 1990. Levamisole and fluorouracil for adjuvant therapy of resected colon carcinoma. *New England Journal of Medicine* 322: 352-8.

Mohiuddin M, and Marks G. 1991. High dose preoperative irradiation for cancer of the rectum, 1976-1988. *International Journal of Radiation Oncology, Biology, Physics* 20: 37-43.

Napolean B, Pujol B, Berger F, et al. 1991. Accuracy of endosonography in the staging of rectal cancer treated by radiotherapy. *British Journal of Surgery* 78: 785-788.

National Institutes of Health. 16 April 1990. Adjuvant Therapy for Patients with Colon and Rectum Cancer. *NIH Consensus Statement Online* 8 (4): 1-25.

Nicholls RJ, York Mason A, Morson BC, Dixon AK, and Fry IK. 1982. The clinical staging of rectal cancer. *British Journal of Surgery* 71: 787-90.

Nogueras JJ, and Jagelman DG. 1993. Principles of surgical resection. Influence of surgical technique on treatment outcome. *Surgical Clinics of North America* 73: 103-116.

O'Connell MJ, Martenson JA, Wiand HS, et al. 1994. Improving adjuvant therapy for rectal cancer by combining protracted-infusion fluorouracil with radiation therapy after curative surgery. *New England Journal of Medicine* 331: 502-507.

O'Connell MJ, Mailliard JA, Kahn MJ, Macdonald JS, Haller DG, Mayer RJ, and Wieand HS. 1997. Controlled trial of fluorouracil and low-dose leucovorin given for 6 months as postoperative adjuvant therapy for colon cancer. *Journal of Clinical Oncology* 15: 246-50.

Pahlman L, and Glimelius B. 1995. The value of adjuvant radio(chemo)therapy for rectal cancer. *European Journal of Cancer* 31A: 1347-50.

Parker GA, Lawrence W Jr, Horsley JS III, et al. 1989. Intraoperative ultrasound of the liver affects operative decision making. *Annals of Surgery* 209: 569-77.

Parker SL, Tong T, Bolden S, and Wingo PA. 1996. Cancer Statistics, 1996. *CA - A Cancer Journal for Clinicians* 46: 5-27.

Patchett SE, Mulcahy HE, and O'Donoghue DP. 1993. Colonoscopy surveillance after curative resection for colorectal cancer. *British Journal of Surgery* 80: 1330-1332.

Pedersen IK, Burchart F, Roikajaer O, and Baden H. 1994. Resection of liver metastases from colorectal cancer. Indications and results. *Diseases of the Colon and Rectum* 37: 1078-1082.

Petrelli N, Douglass HO, Herrera L, et al. 1989. The modulation of fluorouracil with leucovorin in metastatic colorectal carcinoma: a prospective randomized phase III trial. *Journal of Clinical Oncology* 7: 1419-1426.

Petrelli N, Herrera L, Rustrum Y, et al. 1987. A prospective randomized trial of 5-fluorouracil versus 5-fluorouracil and high-dose leucovorin versus 5-fluorouracil and methotrexate in previously untreated patients with advanced colorectal carcinoma. *Journal of Clinical Oncology* 5: 1559-1565.

Poon MA, O'Connell MJ, Moertel CG, et al. 1989. Biochemical modulation of fluorouracil: evidence of significant improvement of survival and quality of life in patients with advanced colorectal carcinoma. *Journal of Clinical Oncology* 7: 1407-1417.

Rothenberg ML, Eckardt JR, Kuhn JG, et al. 1996. Phase II trial of irinotecan in patients with progressive or rapidly recurrent colorectal cancer. *Journal of Clinical Oncology* 14: 1128-1135.

Rougier P, Laplanche A, Huguier M, et al. 1992. Hepatic arterial infusion of floxuridine in patients with liver metastases from colorectal carcinoma: long-term results of a prospective randomized trial. *Journal of Clinical Oncology* 10: 22-28.

Safi F, Link KH, and Beger HG. 1993. Is follow-up of colorectal cancer patients worthwhile? *Diseases of the Colon and Rectum* 36: 636-644.

Saitoh N, Okui K, Sarashina H, et al. 1986. Evaluation of echographic diagnosis of rectal cancer using intrarectal ultrasonic examination. *Diseases of the Colon and Rectum* 29 (4): 234-42.

Scheele J, Stangl R, and Altendorg-Hormann A. 1990. Hepatic metastases from colorectal carcinoma: impact of surgical resection on the natural history. *British Journal of Surgery* 77: 1241-1246.

Scheele J, Stangl R, Altendorf-Hofmann A, and Gall FP. 1991. Indicators of prognosis after hepatic resection for colorectal secondaries. *Surgery* 110: 13-29.

Scholefield JH, and Northover JM. 1995. Surgical management of rectal cancer. *British Journal of Surgery* 82 (6): 745-8.

Sener SF, Imperato JP, Chmiel J, et al. 1989. The use of cancer registry data to study preoperative carcinoembryonic antigen level as an indicator of survival in colorectal cancer. *Cancer* 39: 51-57.

Shank B, Dershaw DD, Carabelli J, et al. 1990. A prospective study of the accuracy of preoperative computed tomographic staging of patients with biopsy-proven rectal carcinoma. *Diseases of the Colon and Rectum* 33: 285-90.

Slanetz CA, Herter FP, and Grinnell RS. 1972. Anterior resection versus abdominoperineal resection for cancer of the rectum and rectosigmoid. *American Journal of Surgery* 123: 110-117.

Staniunas R, and Schoetz DJ. 1993. Extended resection for carcinoma of colon and rectum. *Surgical Clinics of North America* 73: 117-129.

Steele G. 1993. Standard postoperative monitoring of patients after primary resection of colon and rectum cancer. *Cancer Supplemental* 71: 4225-4235.

Steele G, Bleday R, Mayer RJ, et al. 1991. A prospective evaluation of hepatic resection for colorectal carcinoma metastases to the liver: gastrointestinal tumor study group protocol 6584. *Journal of Clinical Oncology* 9: 1105-22.

Stein BL, and Coller JA. 1993. Management of malignant colorectal polyps. *Surgical Clinics of North America* 73: 47-66.

Steinberg SM, Barkin JS, Kaplan RS, et al. 1986. Prognostic indicators of colon tumors: the Gastrointestinal Tumor Study Group experience. *Cancer* 57: 1866-1870.

Sullivan BA, McKinnis R, and Laufman LR. 1995. Quality of life in patients with metastatic colorectal cancer receiving chemotherapy: a randomized, double-blind trial comparing 5-FU versus 5-FU with leucovorin. *Pharmacotherapy* 15: 600-607.

Tartter PI, Slater G, Papatestas AE, et al. 1984. The prognostic significance of elevated serum alkaline phosphatase levels preoperatively in patients with carcinoma of the colon and rectum. *Surgery, Gynecology and Obstetrics* 158: 569-571.

Taylor I. 1996. Liver metastases from colorectal cancer: lessons from past and present clinical studies. *British Journal of Surgery* 456-460.

Theoni RF, Moss AA, Schnyder P, and Margulis AR. 1981. Detection and staging of primary rectal and rectosigmoid cancer by computed tomography. *Radiology* 141: 135-8.

Thomas PR, and Lindblad AS. 1988. Adjuvant postoperative radiotherapy and chemotherapy in rectal carcinoma: a review of the Gastrointestinal Tumor Study Group experience. *Radiotherapy and Oncology* 13: 245-252.

Vignati P, and Robert PL. 1993. Preoperative evaluation and postoperative surveillance for patients with colorectal carcinoma. *Surgical Clinics of North America* 73: 67-84.

Wagman LD, Kemeny MM, Leong L, Terz JJ, Hill R, et al. 1990. A prospective randomized evaluation of the treatment of colorectal cancer metastatic to the liver. *Journal of Clinical Oncology* 8: 1885-1893.

Waizer A, Zitron S, Ben-Baruch D, Baniel J, Wolloch Y, and Dintsman M. 1989. Comparative study for preoperative staging of rectal cancer. *Diseases of the Colon and Rectum* 32: 53-6.

Willett CG, Compton CC, Shellito PC, et al. 1994. Selection factors for local excision or abdominoperineal resection of early stage rectal cancer. *Cancer* 73: 2716-2720.

Winawer SJ, Fletcher RH, Miller L, Godlee F, Stolar MH, et al. 1997. Colorectal cancer screening: clinical guidelines and rationale. *Gastroenterology* 112: 594-642.

Wolmark N, Rockett H, Fisher B, et al. 1993. The benefit of leucovorin-modulated fluorouracil as postoperative adjuvant therapy for primary colon cancer: results from National Surgical Adjuvant Breast and Bowel Project protocol C-03. *Journal of Clinical Oncology* 11: 1879-1887.

Wolmark N, Rockette H, Mamounas EP, Petrelli N, et al. 1996. The relative efficacy of 5-FU + leucovorin (FU-LV), 5-FU+Levamisole (FU-LEV), and 5-FU+leucovorin+levamisole (percentFU-LV-LEV) in patients with Dukes' B and C carcinoma of the colon. First report of NSABP C-04. *Proceedings of ASCO* 15 (460): 205.

RECOMMENDED QUALITY INDICATORS FOR COLORECTAL CANCER TREATMENT

The following apply to men and women age 18 and over who have colorectal cancer.

Indicator	Quality of Evidence	Literature	Benefits	Comments
Diagnosis				
1. Patients who have undergone surgical resection for colon or rectal cancer should have documentation in the chart that colonoscopy or barium enema with sigmoidoscopy was offered within the preceding 12 months.	II-2, III	Vignati and Roberts 1993; Isler et al., 1987	Promote complete cure.	Identifies synchronous lesions so that surgery can be appropriately modified. Between 2% and 7% of patients with colon cancer have a synchronous lesion.
Treatment				
2. Patients diagnosed with a malignant polyp should be offered a wide surgical resection within 6 weeks if any of the following are true: a. the colonoscopy report states that the polyp was not completely excised; b. the margins are positive; c. lymphatic or venous invasion is present; d. histology is grade 3 or poorly differentiated.	II-2, III	Stein and Coller 1993; Bond, 1993	Promote complete cure.	Offers option of curative treatment for persons at high risk of developing recurrent or metastatic disease. Adverse histologic features predict 40-50% rate of recurrence or metastases.
3. Patients with a malignant polyp treated with polypectomy alone should be offered colonoscopy within 6 months of the polypectomy.	III	Bond, 1993	Decrease risk of recurrence.	Ensures that all of the carcinoma has been excised. American College of Gastroenterology recommendation.

Indicator	Quality of Evidence	Literature	Benefits	Comments
4. Patients who are diagnosed with colon cancer and do not have metastatic disease[1] should be offered a wide resection with anastamosis[2] within 6 weeks of diagnosis.	II-2, III	CancerNet 3/97, Haskell 1995; Nogueras and Jagelman et al., 1993; Staniunas and Schoetz 1993;McGlone et al., 1982; Gall et al., 1987	Decrease mortality.	Surgical resection is the only curative treatment.

5. Patients who undergo a wide surgical resection should have "negative margins" noted on the most recent final pathology report or have documentation that they were offered a repeat resection if they meet either of the following criteria:
   a. Stage I colon cancer;[3]
   b. Stage II or III colon cancer[4] that is not invading into other organs (not a T4 lesion[5]).
	II-2, III	Haskell1995; Nogueras and Jagelman, et al., 1993	Decrease risk of recurrence.	Ensures adequate surgical therapy. Risk of recurrence is higher with positive margins.

106

Indicator	Quality of Evidence	Literature	Benefits	Comments
6. Patients with Stage III colon cancer who have undergone a surgical resection should be offered adjuvant chemotherapy[6] within 6 weeks of surgery and not before 21 days after surgery with a published 5-FU-containing regimen.	I, II-2, III	The Medical Letter 1996, Moertel, 1994; Moertel et al., 1990; Laurie et al., 1989; Moertel et al., 1995; NIH 1990; Wolmark et al., 1993; IMPA of Colon Cancer Trials, 1995; O'Connell, et al., 1997; Haller, et al., 1996; Wolmark, et al., 1996	Decreases the risk of recurrence.	Randomized controlled trials have demonstrated approximately a 30% reduction in the overall mortality for patients with Stage III colon cancer treated with 5-FU and levamisole or 5-FU and leucovorin.
7. Patients who are diagnosed with rectal cancer that appears clinically to be Stage I, should be offered one of the following surgical resections within 6 weeks of diagnosis: • low anterior resection; • abdominal perineal resection; • full-thickness local excision.	II-2, III	Butcher Jr., 1971; Malt and Nundy 1974; Slanetz et al., 1972; Mayo and Cullen, 1960; Mayo C et al., 1958; Balsley I and Fenger, 1973; Heald and Ryall 1986;Minsky 1995;, Buess, 1995; Scholefield, 1995; Heimann, et al., 1992; Bailey, et al., 1992; Willett et al., 1994	Offers option of curative treatment.	Surgical resection is the only curative treatment.
8. Patients who are diagnosed with rectal cancer that appears clinically to be Stage II or III, should be offered one of the following surgical resections within 6 weeks of diagnosis: • low anterior resection; • abdominal perineal resection.	II-2, III	Butcher Jr., 1971; Malt and Nundy, 1974; Slanetz et al., 1972,; Mayo and Cullen,1960; Mayo et al., 1958; Balsley and Fenger, 1973;	Promotes complete cure.	Surgical resection is the only curative treatment.

	Indicator	Quality of Evidence	Literature	Benefits	Comments
9.	Patients who undergo a wide surgical resection should have "negative margins" noted on the most recent final pathology report or have documentation that they were offered a repeat resection if they meet either of the following criteria: a. Stage I rectal cancer; b. Stage II or III rectal cancer that is not invading into other organs (not a T4 lesion).	II-2, III	Butcher, 1971; Malt and Nundy, 1974; Slanetz et al., 1972; Mayo and Cullen,1960; Mayo, et al., 1958; Balsley and Fenger, 1973; Heald and Ryall, 1986; Minsky, 1995; Buess, 1995; Scholefield, 1995; Heimann et al., 1992; Bailey,et al., 1992; Willett, et al., 1994;	Promotes complete cure.	Ensures adequate surgical therapy. Risk of recurrence is higher with positive margins.
10.	Patients with Stage II and III rectal cancer (defined pathologically) who undergo surgical resection should be offered one of the following treatments (*this indicator only applies to patients who have had a surgical resection*): • postoperative radiation therapy of 45-55 Gy to the pelvis with chemotherapy containing 5-FU to begin not sooner than 4 weeks after surgery and not more than 12 weeks after surgery; • preoperative radiation therapy to the pelvis to begin not more than 6 weeks after diagnosis; • preoperative radiation therapy with chemotherapy containing 5-FU to begin not more than 6 weeks after diagnosis.	I, II-2, III	Heald,1986; Gerard, et al., 1988; Thomas and Lindblad, 1988; Fisher et al., 1988; Mohiuddin, 1991, Thomas and Lindblad, 1988; The Medical Letter, 1996; Pahlman, 1995; Freedman, 1995; Krook, et al., 1991; GTS Group, 1992; Moertel, 1994; GTS Group, 1984; O'Conell et al., 1994	Decreases risk of recurrence.	NIH Consensus Conference recommendation (1990).

	Indicator	Quality of Evidence	Literature	Benefits	Comments
11.	Patients receiving 5-FU chemotherapy should have a CBC checked not more than 48 hours prior to the first dose in each cycle.	II-2, III	The Medical Letter 1996; Erlichman, 1988; Doroshow, et al., 1990; Petrelli et al, 1989; Petrelli et al., 1987; Leichman et al., 1995; Poon et al., 1989; Moertel et al., 1990; Laurie et al., 1989; Wolmark et al., 1993; IMPA of Colon Cancer Trials 1995	Avoid excess morbidity and mortality from chemotherapy toxicity.	Most common dose-limiting side-effect of the five-day daily 5-FU fast infusion is neutropenia.
12.	Patients should not receive 5-FU chemotherapy if any of the following are documented in the past 2 days: a. WBC < 2,000; b. stomatitis that prevents them from eating; c. diarrhea of seven or more stools a day.	II-2, III	The Medical Letter 1996; Erlichman, 1988; Doroshow, et al., 1990; Petrelli et al, 1989; Petrelli et al., 1987; Leichman et al., 1995; Poon et al., 1989; Moertel et al., 1990; Laurie et al., 1989; Wolmark et al., 1993; IMPA of Colon Cancer Trials 1995	Avoid excess morbidity and mortality from chemotherapy toxicity.	Grade 3 or 4 toxicity is an indication to hold chemotherapy and reduce the dosage.
Follow-up					
13.	Patients with Stages I, II, and III colorectal cancer should receive a visit with a physician for a history and physical where colorectal cancer is addressed in the assessment and plan at least every 6 months for 3 years after initial treatment.	II-2, III	Vignati and Robert, 1993; Safi et al., 1993; Steele, 1993; Beart et al., 1983; Deveney et al., 1984	Decrease mortality.	Identifies patients with recurrent disease or a metachronous cancer early . 85% of colorectal cancers recur in the first 3 years.

109

	Indicator	Quality of Evidence	Literature	Benefits	Comments
14.	Patients with Stages I, II, and III colorectal cancer should receive colonoscopy or double contrast barium enema within a year of curative surgery if it did not occur within 12 months preoperatively.	II-2, III	Winawer et al., 1997; Lautenbach et al., 1994; Barlow and Thompson 1993; Patchett et al., 1993	Decrease mortality.	Identifies patients with recurrent disease or a metachronous cancer early. 85% of colorectal cancers recur in the first 3 years.
15	Patients with Stages I, II, and III colorectal cancer should receive colonoscopy or double contrast barium enema three years after surgery and every five years thereafter.	II-2, III	Winawer et al., 1997; Lautenbach et al., 1994; Barlow and Thompson, 1993, Patchett, et al., 1993	Decrease risk of recurrence.	Identifies patients with recurrent disease or a metachronous cancer early. 85% of colorectal cancers recur in the first 3 years.

110

Definitions and Examples

[1] Metastatic disease - A patient shall be considered to have metastatic disease if a chest x-ray, CT scan of the abdomen, adominal ultrasound, bone scan, or plain films of the bones show evidence of metastatic disease as follows:

    a. Chest X-ray - nodules or masses
    b. CT scan of the abdomen - nodules or masses in the liver
    c. Abdominal Ultrasound - hypoechoic lesions in the liver
    d. Bone Scan - increased uptake
    e. Plain Films - lytic or blastic bone lesions.

[2] Wide Resection with Anastamosis - evidence of wide resection will be obtained from the pathology report as follows: The surgical specimen must include the tumor with at least 2cm of bowel on either side, and there must be lymph nodes present.

[3] To be clinically Stage I, all of the following criteria must be met:

    a. On digital rectal exam, tumor is not fixed to pelvis.
    b. If endorectal ultrasound is performed there is no transmural penetration of tumor.
    c. No evidence of metastatic disease.

[4] To be clinically Stage II or III, all of the following criteria must be met:

    a. On digital rectal exam, tumor is fixed to pelvis.
    b. If endorectal ultrasound is performed there is transmural penetration of tumor
    c. No evidence of metastatic disease.

[5] T4 lesion - tumor penetrates the visceral peritoneum or invades other organs or structures.

[6] Adjuvant chemotherapy: Acceptable 5-FU containing regimens include the following:

5-FU 300-600mg/m^2 intravenous, daily for 5 days repeated every 28 days OR weekly, plus Levamisole 50mg orally 3 times a day for 3 days every 2 weeks OR Leucovorin 20-500mg/m2 intravenous with each dose of 5-FU.

Quality of Evidence Codes:

I	Randomized controlled trials
II-1	Nonrandomized controlled trials
II-2	Cohort or case analysis
II-3	Multiple time series
III	Opinions or descriptive

6. HIV DISEASE

Steven Asch, MD, MPH

Six practice guidelines (Carpenter et al., 1996; NIH Draft Principles, 1997; NIH Draft Guidelines, 1997; AHCPR, 1994; MMWR, 1988; MMWR, 1995) and five reviews (Bozette and Asch, 1995; Hopkins HIV Report, 1997; Jewett and Hecht, 1993; Richards, Kovacs, and Luft, 1995; Simonds, Hughes, Feinberg, and Navin, 1995) provided the background material in developing quality indicators for HIV disease. We also performed MEDLINE searches of the medical literature from 1993 to 1996 to supplement these references.

IMPORTANCE

HIV/AIDS is a devastating medical and public health problem in the United States and throughout the world. Approximately one million individuals are estimated to have HIV infection in the U.S, although the number of new cases may be leveling off (MMWR, 1996). In the U.S., HIV disease is currently the leading cause of death among young men, and the fastest-rising cause of death among young women. Estimates of the number of new U.S. AIDS cases per year range from 43,000 to 93,000. The majority of AIDS cases in the U.S. are in gay/bisexual men (63%) or intravenous drug users (23%), most of whom live in large metropolitan areas. However, an increase in AIDS incidence in suburban and rural parts of the country is already being seen and is expected to continue (Cohn et al., 1994).

Although the reach of the epidemic is broad, recent improvements in HIV treatment show great promise. New, effective regimens are available to decrease viral loads (Markowitz et al., 1995; Danner et al., 1995; Collier et al., 1996; Kitchen et al., 1995) and prevent opportunistic infections (Simonds et al., 1995; Richards et al., 1995; Ostroff, 1995). Because of these advances, HIV disease has joined conditions such as diabetes, asthma, and atherosclerotic disease as a chronic, manageable illness (Benjamin, 1990). With timely and effective care, many Americans infected with HIV can expect to live full, productive lives for years and even decades (Osmond et al., 1994; Muñoz et al. 1989; Sheppard et al., 1993; Moss and Bacchetti, 1989).

Because the care of HIV-positive patients is so complex, we have concentrated our quality indicators on the following common and important areas: (1) screening and prevention of opportunistic infections and other diagnostic testing, (2) CD4 and viral load monitoring, and (3) antiretroviral therapy. Screening and diagnosis of HIV infection itself and prevention of its spread are covered elsewhere (see the Preventive Care chapter for the General Medicine Panel), and treatment of opportunistic infections is not covered at all. Screening for cervical cancer in HIV patients is also covered elsewhere (see Chapter 3), as is screening for TB infection (see Preventive Care chapter for the General Medicine Panel). Prevention of active TB disease is covered in this chapter.

SCREENING AND PREVENTION

HIV-infected patients are at high risk for developing a wide variety of opportunistic infections. As a result, they benefit from screening tests to detect the presence of the infection, and in some cases, presumptive therapy to prevent the opportunistic infection once immune function drops below certain threshold levels. This section discusses the evidence on screening and prevention for the following opportunistic infections: (1) Pnuemocystis carinii pneumonia (PCP), (2) Tuberculosis (TB), (3) Toxoplasmosis encephalitis (TE), (4) Mycobacterium avium complex (MAC), (5) Pneumococcal pneumonia, (6) Cytomegalovirus retinitis (CMV), and (7) Syphilis.

Pnuemocystis Carinii Pneumonia (PCP)

PCP is the most common serious opportunistic infection among HIV patients. Prospective follow-up of a cohort of 2,627 HIV-infected men showed it to be the most common AIDS-defining condition in the absence of prophylaxis. Over 42 percent of the 873 men whose infection had progressed to AIDS had PCP. The incidence of PCP decreased in the early 1990s, most likely due to increasing use of effective primary prophylaxis (Simonds et al., 1995; Muñoz, 1989). Without prophylaxis, cumulative incidence of PCP infection rises dramatically as the CD4 count drops, nearing 20 percent for those with CD4 counts under 200. Unexplained prolonged fever (temperature over 100°F for more than two weeks) and oral candidiasis are also associated with the development of pneumonia (Phair, 1990). Nine RCTs using some combination of these criteria and other AIDS-defining illnesses have shown the following

114

regimens to reduce the incidence of PCP: 1) TMP/SMX (single strength or double strength at least three times per week), 2) Dapsone (100 mg/day), 3) aerosolized pentamidine (300 mg four times per month), 4) Dapsone (50 mg/day) plus pyrimethamine (50 mg/week) and leucovorin (25 mg/week), 5) Dapsone (200 mg/week) (Simonds et al., 1995; Fischl, 1988; Leoung, 1990; Slavin, 1992; Schneider, 1992; Hardy, 1992; Girad, 1993; Mallolas, 1993; Opravil, 1995; Bozzette and Asch, 1995). Guidelines from the Centers for Disease Control (CDC) and others recommend prophylactic therapy for all patients with nadir CD4 counts less than 200, previous PCP, unexplained fever, or oral candidiasis (MMWR, 1991; MMWR, 1995; NIH Draft Guidelines, 1997). We have reproduced those recommendations as a quality indicator (Indicator 1), but have left out the indication of unexplained fever due to potential difficulties in abstracting this information from the medical record.

Tuberculosis (TB)

HIV-positive patients are both more likely to have been infected with TB before contracting HIV and to develop active TB once HIV infection is established. Co-infected patients have a ten percent annual risk of developing active TB (Selwyn, 1989). Although no randomized trials are available, experts usually recommend screening with some combination of history, PPD and anergy testing, and chest x-ray. One study (Jordan, 1991) supports treatment of latent disease for all HIV patients, regardless of screening results. However, most experts now recommend isoniazid therapy if the PPD is greater than 5 mm inuration in the absence of active disease, or if the patient has been recently exposed to someone with active disease (AHCPR, 1994; Hopkins HIV Report, 1997) (Indicator 2).

Toxoplasmosis Encephalitis (TE)

TE occurs in ten to 50 percent of patients who are seropositive for antibodies to *Toxoplasma gondii* and who have CD4 counts less than 100. The relative risk for developing the disease in seropositives as compared to seronegatives is 27 (Oskenhendler, 1994). Two RCTs and one observational trial with seropositives show that pyrimethamine and the combination of dapsone and pyramethamine are effective in preventing TE. One RCT showed it to be ineffective, but many of the patients in that trial were on concurrent PCP prophylaxis (Jacobson, 1994; Girad, 1993; Clotet, 1991; Clotet, 1992;

Bachmeyer, 1994). Observational and laboratory data suggest that anti-PCP regimens containing TMP/SMX are also effective (Richards et al., 1995). Expert groups have recommended that all patients be tested for toxoplasmosis antibodies upon diagnosis (MMWR, 1995). Seropositive patients with CD4 counts above 100 should be counseled on avoidance of exposure and those with CD4 counts under 100 should be offered one of the above regimes. We have developed quality indicators to reflect the chemoprophylactic recommendations (Indicator 3) and the screening test recomendations (Indicator 4).

Mycobaterium Avium Complex (MAC)

Disseminated MAC is a late-stage complication of HIV infection, eventually affecting 15 to 25 percent of patients with CD4 counts less than 100 (Horsberg, 1991; Nightingale, 1992). Two RCTs of rifabutin in patients with CD4 counts less than 200 showed a 50 percent reduction in the incidence of MAC disease. One of these two trials also showed a mortality benefit (Nightingale, 1993). An RCT of clarithromycin showed an effect of similar magnitude on the incidence of bacteremia for patients with CD4 counts less than 100. This study also showed a positive effect on prevention of mortality (Pierce et al., 1996). Most of the beneficial effect of prophylactic regimens occurs in patients with CD4 counts below 50. Another RCT showed weekly azithromycin to be more effective in preventing disease than rifabutin (Havlir et al., 1996). The results of this trial, and rifabutin's unfavorable drug interactions, have led to a preference for clarithromycin or azithromycin. Recent CDC recommendations (MMWR, 1997) call for any one of the three therapies for patients with CD4 counts of less than 50 (Indicator 5).

Pneumococcal Pneumonia

Vaccination of HIV patients with capsular antigens of multiple strains of pneumococcus induces levels of antibodies thought to be protective for pneumonia, however no clinical trials have directly examined the vaccine's efficacy in preventing disease in this population. The CDC has nonetheless recommended its use in all HIV patients as early as possible so as to promote immune response (MMWR, 1995) (Indicator 6).

Cytomegalovirus (CMV) retinitis

CMV retinitis is another late-stage complication of HIV disease. Patients with CD4 counts less than 100 have a 21 percent probability of developing CMV infection within two years, usually retinitis (Gallant, 1992, 1994). While one study has shown that oral ganciclovir reduces the risk of CMV (Spector, 1997), the therapy is expensive and not strongly recommended for primary prophylaxis. However, treatment of known CMV retinitis prevents progression to blindness (Masur, 1996) and guidelines from AHCPR and others support at least annual screening fundoscopy for all patients with CD4 counts less than 100 (AHCPR, 1994; Masur, 1996) (Indicator 7). The CDC guidelines also recommend fundoscopic screening, although without specifying a CD4 threshold (MMWR, 1995).

Syphilis

Coinfection with syphilis occurs in one to ten percent of HIV patients (Quinn et al., 1990; 1996; Telzak et al., 1993; Lurie et al., 1995). The virulence of syphilis is greater in HIV-positive patients and the positive predictive value of the VDRL or RPR tests in HIV, despite early doubts, appears to be high (Jewett and Hecht, 1993). Several trials of treatment of HIV patients screened positive for syphilis have shown efficacy in reducing titers (Malone et al., 1995) and experts recommend screening and treatment with penicillin for HIV positive patients (MMWR, 1988, AHCPR, 1994) (Indicators 8 and 9).

DIAGNOSIS

The initial diagnosis of HIV disease usually depends on the measurement of HIV antibody status, except in the rare instance of diagnosed symptomatic primary HIV. In addition, untested patients with unexplained symptoms of immunosuppression (e.g., fever, thrush) should also be offered testing. We have not included a diagnostic indicator for symptom- and condition-based HIV testing because of the difficulty in determining from the medical record whether such symptoms were unexplained.

Once an initial diagnosis of HIV is established, certain diagnostic tests are universally recommended. Guidelines dictate the measurement of a complete blood count, as both a baseline for following potential hematologic side effects of antiretroviral treatment and a screen for HIV complications such as idiopathic thrombocytopenic purpura (Hopkins, 1997, AHCPR, 1994) (Indicator 10). Both blood CD4 counts and plasma HIV RNA viral load measurement independently predict probability of progression to AIDS and mortality (AHCPR, 1994; Katzenstein et al., 1996; Mellors et al., 1997; O'Brien et al., 1996; MMWR, 1995; O'Brien, 1996; Jurriaans, 1994; Saksela, 1995; Enger, 1996; Dickover, 1994; McIntosh, 1996; Mofenson, 1997; Shearere, 1997; Stein, 1992). While no study has directly examined whether a program of measuring CD4 and viral load itself prevents progression, expert panels are in universal agreement that they should be measured at initial diagnosis for staging (Indicator 10). In order to quickly detect eligibility for antiretroviral therapy, patients with CD4 counts over 500 should have the same tests repeated at least every six months, and patients with CD4 counts less than 500 should have them measured every three months (Indicator 11 and 12). Once the patient is taking antiretrovirals, experts agree that CD4 count and viral load should be measured quarterly. In addition, quarterly screens for side effects of antiretroviral therapy should include CBC to detect hematologic complications (Hopkins, 1997; AHCPR, 1994) (Indicator 13). Other drug-specific screens for side effects are not covered here.

TREATMENT

There are now 11 drugs approved for treatment of HIV infection. More are under development. These drugs fall into three broad classes:

- Nucleoside reverse transcriptase inhibitors (NRTIs): zidovudine (AZT, ZDV), didanosine (Videx, ddI), zalcitabine (HIVID, ddC), stavudine (Zerit, d4T), and lamuvidine (Epivir, 3TC).
- Protease inhibitors: saquinavir (Invirase), ritonovir (Norvir), indinavir (Crixivan) and nelfinavir (Viracept).
- Nonnucleoside reverse transcriptase inhibitors (NNRTIs): nevirapin (Viramune) and delavirdien (Rescriptor).

The rapid expansion of the chemotheraputic armamentarium has generated confusion about when to start therapy and what is the ideal regimen. Many regimens have been shown to reduce viral loads: two NRTIs with a protease inhibitor, two NRTIs with an NNRTI, two NRTIs alone, ddI alone, d4T alone. As discussed above, plasma HIV RNA viral loads correlate strongly with clinical progression of the disease. Perhaps the most potent combination in reducing viral loads would include two NRTIs and a protease inhibitor (NIH Draft Guidelines, 1997).

Trials that evaluate clinical endpoints rather than the surrogate marker of viral loads are rare and more likely to evaluate the older agents. Initial placebo-controlled studies of monotherapy with ZDV in antiretroviral-naive patients showed a delay in progression to AIDS but only a debatable survival benefit (Fischl et al., 1990; Volberding et al., 1990). Since then, the following combinations have been shown in RCTs to be superior to ZDV monotherapy in preventing disease progression or death: ZDV/DDI, DDI alone, ZDV/zalcitabine (Eron et al., 1995; Hammer et al. 1996; Collier et al., 1996; Schooley et al., 1996; D'Aquila et al., 1996). These effects were most pronounced in patients with CD4 counts between 200 and 500. Adding protease inhibitors to the regimens of patients who have already taken NRTIs has been shown to reduce progression and death, particularly in patients with advanced disease (Carpenter et al., 1996).

Experts are divided into two camps with regard to the initiation of therapy. One advocates using the most potent antiretroviral regimen first, in all patients, early in the course of the infection. The recent preliminary report from the NIH consensus panel (NIH Draft Guidelines, 1997) supports this position. The other camp reserves the most potent therapy for those with higher pretreatment progression risk, or for those who progress despite less potent therapy. We believe that both approaches are defensible with current clinical trial evidence.

In the proposed quality indicator we have concentrated on areas of agreement (Indicator 14). We included any treatment regimen that has been shown to reduce viral load more effectively than ZDV monotherapy. In addition, we have used the more conservative combined CD4 and viral load cut-points for initiation of therapy, as proposed by the International AIDS Society Panel in 1996 (Carpenter et al., 1996). This indicator would not penalize providers or plans who take the more aggressive approach, but would identify care that both camps consider inadequate.

Protease inhibitors have certain drawbacks despite high antiretroviral activity. One of them is drug interaction with commonly prescribed antihistamines, antibiotics, and promotilic agents. We recommend an indicator that proscribes those drug combinations (Indicator 15).

119

FOLLOW-UP

Many experts recommend that viral load be measured within a few weeks of changes in antiretroviral therapy in order to gauge the response, though the threshold of response for determining successful or failed therapy is a matter of some debate (NIH Draft Guidelines, 1997; Hopkins HIV Report, 1997) (Indicator 16).

REFERENCES

Bachmeyer C, et al. 1994. Pyrimethamine as primary prophylaxis of toxoplasmic encephalitits in patients infected with Human Immunodeficiency Virus: open study. *Clinical Infectious Diseases* 18: 479-80.

Benjamin AE. 1990. *Chronic illness and a continuum of care for persons with HIV-related illnesses.* In: AHCPR conference proceedings of community-based care of persons with AIDS: developing a research agenda. U.S. Department of Health and Human Services, Minnesota.

Bozette SA, and Asch SM. 1995. Developing quality review criteria from standards of care for HIV Disease: a framework. *Journal of Acquired Immune Defense Syndromes and Human Retrovirology* 8 (1): S45-S52.

Carpenter C, Fischl M, Hammer S, et al. 1996. Consensus Statement — Antiretroviral therapy for HIV infection in 1996: Recommendations of an international panel. *Journal of the American Medical Association* 276: 146-154.

Clotet B, et al. 1992. Cerebral toxoplasmosis and prophylaxis for pnemoncystis carinii pnemonia. *Archives of Internal Medicine* 117 (2): 169.

Clotet B, et al. 1991. Correspondence. *AIDS* 5 (5): 601-602.

Cohn SE, Klein JD, Mohr JE, van der Horst CM, and Weber DJ. 1994. The geography of AIDS: patterns of urban and rural migration. *Southern Medical Journal* 87 (6): 599-606.

Collier AC, Coombs RW, Schoenfeld DA, et al. 1996. Treatment of human immunodeficiency virus infection with saquinavir, zidovudine, and zalcitabine. AIDS Clinical Trials Group. *New England Journal of Medicine* 334 (16): 1011-7.

Danner SA, Carr A, Leonard JM, et al. 1995. A short-term study of the safety, pharmacokinetics, and efficacy of ritonavir, an inhibitor of HIV-1 protease. European-Australian Collaborative Ritonavir Study Group. *New England Journal of Medicine* 333 (23): 1528-33.

D'Aquila RT, Hughes MD, Johnson VA, et al. 1996. Nevirapine, Zidovudine, and Didanosine compared with Zidovudine and Didanosine in patients with HIV-1 infection. *Annals of Internal Medicine* 124 (12): 1019-1030.

Dickover RE, Dillon M, Gillette SG, et al. 1994. Rapid increase in load of human immunodeficiency virus Correlate with Early Disease Progression and Loss of CD4 Cells in Vertically Infected Infants. *Journal of Infectious Diseases* 170: 1279-84.

Enger C, et al. 1996. Survival from early, intermediate and late stages of HIV Infection. *Journal of the American Medical Association* 275: 1329-34.

Eron J, Benoit S, Jemsek J, et al. 1995. Treatment with lamivudine, zidovudine, or both in HIV-positive patients with 200 to 500 CD4+ cells per cubic millimeter. *New England Journal of Medicine* 333: 1662-1669.

Fischl MA, Dickinson GD, and La Voie L. 1988. Safety and efficaacy of sulfamethoazole and trimethoprim chemoprophylaxis for pneumocystis carinii pneumonia in AIDS. *Journal of the American Medical Association* 259 (8): 1185-1189.

Fischl MA, Richman DD, Hansen N, et al. 1990. The Safety and efficacy of Zidovudine (AZT) in the treatment of subjects with mildly symptomatic Human Immunodeficiency Virus type 1 (HIV) infection. *Annals of Internal Medicine* 112: 727-737.

Gallant JE, Moore RD, Richman DD, Keruly J, and Chaisson RE. December 1992. Incidence and natural history of cytomegalovirus disease in patients with advanced human immunodeficiency virus disease treated with zidovudine. The Zidovudine Epidemiology Study Group. *Journal of Infectious Diseases* 166 (6): 1223-7.

Gallant JE, Moore RD, and Chaisson RE. 1994. Prophylaxis for opportunistic infections in patients with HIV infection [see comments]. *Archives of Internal Medicine* 120 (11): 932-44.

Girard PM, Landman R, Gaudebout C, et al. 1993. Dapsone-Pyrimethamine compared with aerosolized pnetamidine as primary prophylaxis against pnemocystis carinii pneumoia and toxoplasmosis in HIV infection. *New England Journal of Medicine* 328 (21): 1514-1520.

Hammer SM, Katzenstein DA, Hughes MD, et al. 1996. A trial comparing nucleoside monotherapy with combination therapy in HIV-infected adults with CD4 cell counts from 200 to 500 per cubic millimeter. *New England Journal of Medicine* 335: 1081-1090.

Hardy WD, Feiberg J, et al. 1992. A controlled trial of timethoprim-sulfamethoxazole or aerosolized pentamidine for secondary prophylaxis of pneumocystis carinii pneumonia in patients with the acquired immunodeficiency syndrome. *New England Journal of Medicine* 327 (26): 1842-1848.

Havlir DV, Dube MP, Sattler FR, et al. Prophylaxis against disseminated mycobacterium avium complex with weekly azithromycin, daily rifabutin, or both. *New England Journal of Medicine* 335 (6): 392-398.

Hopkins HIV Report. March 1997. Update on HIV Management: Recommendations of the Johns Hopkins University AIDS Service.

Horsburgh CR, et al. 1991. Survival of patients with acquired immune deficiency syndrome and disseminated mycobacterium avium complex infection with and without antimycobacterial chemotherapy. *American Review of Repiratory Disease* 144: 557-559.

Jacobson MA, Besch CL, Child C, Hafner R, Matts JP, Muth K, Wentworth DN, Neaton JD, Abrams D, Rimland D, et al. February 1994. Primary prophylaxis with pyrimethamine for toxoplasmic encephalitis in patients with advanced human immunodeficiency virus disease: results of a randomized trial. *Journal of Infectious Diseases* 169 (2): 384-94.

Jewett JF, and Hecht FM. 1993. Preventive health care for adults with HIV infection. *Journal of the American Medical Association* 269 (9): 1144-53.

Jordan TJ, Lewit EM, and Reichman LB. December 1991. Isoniazid preventive therapy for tuberculosis. Decision analysis considering ethnicity and gender. *American Review of Respiratory Disease* 144 (6): 1357-60.

Jurriaans S, van Gemen B, et al. 1994. The natural history of HIV-1 infection: virus load and Virus Phenotype Independent Determinants of Clinical Course? *Virology* 204: 223-33.

Kitchen VS, Skinner C, Ariyoshi K, et al. 1995. Safety and activity of saquinavir in HIV infection. *Lancet* 345 (8955): 952-5.

Leoung GS, Feigal DW, and Mongomery B. 1990. Aerosolized pentamidine for prophylaxis against pnemocystis carinii pneumonia. *New England Journal of Medicine* 323 (12): 769-775.

Lurie P, Fernandes ME, Hughes V, et al. 1995. Socioeconomic status and risk of HIV-1, syphilis and hepatitis B infection among sex workers in Sao Paulo State, Brazil. *AIDS* 9 (suppl 1): S31-S37.

Mallolas J, Zamora L, Gatell J, et al. 1993. Pimary prophylaxis for pneumoncystis carinii pneumonia: a randomized trial comparing cotrimoxazole, aerosolized pentamidine and dapsone plus pyrimethamine. *AIDS* 7: 59-64.

Malone JL, Wallace MR, Hendrick BB, et al. 1995. Syphilis and neurosyphilis in a Human Immunodeficiency Virus Type-1 seropositive population: evidence for frequent serlogic relapse after therapy. *American Journal of Medicine* 99: 55-63.

Markowitz M, Saag M, Powderly WG, et al. 1995. A preliminary study of ritonavir, an inhibitor of HIV-1 protease, to treat HIV-1 infection. *New England Journal of Medicine* 333 (23): 1534-9.

Masur H, Whitcup SM, Cartwright C, Polis M, and Nussenblatt R. 1996. Advances in the management of AIDS-related cytomegalovirus retinitis. *Archives of Internal Medicine* 125 (2): 126-36.

Mcintosh K, et al. 1996. Age and time related changes in extracellular viral load in children vertically infected by human immunodeficiency virus. *Pediatric Infectious Diseases Journal* 15: 1087-91.

Mellors JW, Munoz A, Giorgi JV, et al. 1997. Plasma viral load and Cd4+ lymphocytes as prognostic markers of HIV-1 infection. *Archives of Internal Medicine* 126: 946-954.

Morbidity and Mortality Weekly Report. 1996. AIDS Rates. *Morbidity and Mortality Weekly Report* 45 (42): 926-7.

Morbidity and Mortality Weekly Report. 1991. Purified Protein Derivative (PPD)-tuberculin anergy and HIV infection: guidelines for anergy testing and management of anergic persons at risk of tuberculosis. *Morbidity and Mortality Weekly Report* 40 (no RR-5): 27-33.

Morbidity and Mortality Weekly Report. 1988. Recommendations for diagnosing and treating syphilis in HIV-infected patients. *Morbitiy and Mortality Weekly Report* 37: 600-608.

Mofenson LM, et al. 1997. The relationship between serum human immunodeficiency Virus type 1 (HIV-1) RNA Level, CD4, Lymphocyte Percent, and Long-Term Mortality Risk in HIV-1 Infected Children. *Journal of Infectious Diseases* 175: 1029-38.

Moss AR, and Bacchetti P. 1989. Natural history of HIV infection [published erratum appears in AIDS 1989 Jul;3(7):following A100]. *AIDS* 3 (2): 55-61.

Munoz A, Wang MC, Bass S, et al. 1989. Acquired immunodeficiency syndrome (AIDS)-free time after human immunodeficiency virus type 1 (HIV-1) seroconversion in homosexual men Multicenter AIDS Cohort Study Group. *American Journal of Epidemiology* 130 (3): 530-9.

Nightingale SD, Byrd LT, Southern PM, et al. 1992. Incidence of mycobacterium avium-intracellalare complex bacteremia in human immunodeficiency virus-positive patients. *Journal of Infectious Diseases* 165: 1082-5.

Nightingale SD, Cameron DW, Gordin FM, et al. 1993. Two controlled trials of rifabutin Prophylaxis against mycobacterium avium complex infection in AIDS. *New England Journal of Medicine* 329: 828-33.

O'Brien TR, Blattner WA, Waters D, et al. 1996. Serum HIV-1 RNA levels and time to development of AIDS in the multicenter hemophilia cohort study. *Journal of the American Medical Association* 276: 105-10.

Opravil M, Hirschel B, and Lazzarin A. 1995. Once-weekly administration of dapsone/pyrimethamine vs. aerosolized pentamidine as combined prophylaxis for pneumocystis carinii pneumonia and toxoplasmis encephalitis in Human Immunodeficiency Virus-infected patients. *Clinical Infectious Diseases* 20: 531-41.

Oskenhendler E, Charreau I, et al. 1994. Toxoplasma gondii infection in advanced HIV infection. *AIDS* 8: 483-487.

Osmond, Charlebois, Lang, Shiboski, and Moss. April 1994. Changes in AIDS
    survivial time in two San Francisco cohorts of homosexual men, 1983 to
    1993. *Journal of the American Medical Association* 271 (14): 1083-1087.

Phair J, Munoz A, Detels R, et al. 1990. The risk of pneumocystis carinii
    pneumonia among men infected with Human Immunodeficiency Virus Type 1.
    New England Journal of Medicine 322 (3): 161-165.

Pierce M, Crampton S, Henry D, et al. 1996. A randomized trial of
    clarithromycin as prophylaxis against disseminated mycobacterium avium
    complex infection in patients with advanced acquired immunodeficiency
    syndrome. *New England Journal of Medicine* 335 (6): 384-391.

Quinn TC, Cannon RO, Glasser D, et al. 1990. The association of syphilis with
    risk of human immunodeficiency virus infection in patients attending
    sexually transmitted disease clinics. *Archives of Internal Medicine* 150:
    1297-1302.

Report of the NIH Panel to Define Principles of Therapy of HIV Infection.
    Draft Guidelines 1997.

Richards FO Jr, Kovacs JA, and Luft BJ. August 1995. Preventing toxoplasmic
    encephalitis in persons infected with human immunodeficiency virus.
    Clinical Infectious Diseases 21 (Suppl 1): S49-56.

Saksela K, Stevens CE, et al. 1995. HIV-1 messenger RNA in peripheral blood
    mononuclear cells as an early marker of risk for progression to AIDS.
    Archives of Internal Medicine 123: 641-48.

Schearer WT, Quinn TC, et al. 1997. Viral load and disease progression in
    infants infected with Humman Immunodeficiency virus type 1. *New England
    Journal of Medicine* 336: 1337.

Schneider M, et al. 1992. A controlled trial of aerosolized pentamidine or
    Trimethoprim-sulfamethoxazole as primary prophylaxis against pnemocystis
    carinii pneumonia in patients with human immunodeficiency virus
    infection. *New England Journal of Medicine* 327 (26): 1836-1841.

Schooley RT, Ramirez-Ronda C, and Lange JM. 1996. Virologic and immunologic
    benefits of initial combination therapy with zidovudine and zalcitabine
    or didanosine compared with zidovudine monotherapy. *Journal of
    Infectious Diseases* 173: 1354-66.

Selwyn PA, Hartel D, Lewis VA, Schoenbaum EE, Vermund SH, Klein RS, Walker AT,
    and Friedland GH. 2 March 1989. A prospective study of the risk of
    tuberculosis among intravenous drug users with human immunodeficiency
    virus infection. *New England Journal of Medicine* 320 (9): 545-50.

Sheppard HW, Lang W, Ascher MS, Vittinghoff E, and Winkelstein W. 1993. The
    characterization of non-progressors: long-term HIV-1 infection with
    stable CD4+ T-cell levels. *AIDS* 7 (9): 1159-66.

Simonds RJ, Hughes WT, Feinberg J, and Navin TR. 1995. Preventing Pneumocystis carinii pneumonia in persons infected with human immunodeficiency virus. *Clinical Infectious Diseases* 21 (Suppl 1): S44-8.

Slavin MA, Hoy JF, Stewart K, et al. 1992. Oral dapsone versus nebulized pentamidine for Pneumocystis carinii pneumonia prophylaxis: an open randomized prospective trial to assess efficacy and haematological toxity. *AIDS* 6: 1169-1174.

Spector SA, McKinley GF, Lalezari JP, et al. 6 June 1996. Oral ganciclovir for the prevention of cytomegalovirus disease inpersons with AIDS. Roche Cooperative Oral Ganciclovir Study Group. *New England Journal of Medicine* 334 (23): 1491-7.

Stein DS, Korvick JA, and Vermund SH. 1992. CD4+ lympocyte cell enumeration for prediction of clinical course of human immunodeficiency virus disease: a review. *Journal of Infectious Diseases* 165: 352-63.

Telzak EE, Chiasson MA, Bevier PJ, et al. 1993. HIV-1 seroconversion in patients with and without genital ulcer disease. *Archives of Internal Medicine* 119 (12): 1181-1186.

US Department of Health and Human Services. January 1994. *Evaluation and Management of Early HIV Infection. Clinical Practice Guideline Number 7.*

USPHS, and IDSA Prevention of Opportunistic Infections Working Group. 1995. USPHS/IDSA guidelines for the prevention of opportunistic infections in persons infected with human immunodeficiency virus. *Morbidity and Mortality Weekly Report* 11: 1-34.

Volberding P, Lagakos S, Koch M, et al. 1990. Zidovudine in asymptomatic human immunodeficiency virus infection: A controlled trial in persons with fewer than 500 CD4-positive cells per cubic millimeter. *New England Journal of Medicine* 322: 941-949.

RECOMMENDED QUALITY INDICATORS FOR HIV DISEASE

The following indicators apply to men and women age 18 and older.

Indicator	Quality of Evidence	Literature	Benefits	Comments
Screening and Prevention				

1. HIV+ patients should be offered PCP prophylaxis[1] within one month of meeting any of the following conditions:
  a. CD4 count dropping below 200;
  b. Thrush;
  c. Completion of active treatment of PCP.
	I
	
	—
	—
	III
		MMWR, 1995; MMWR, 1991; Simonds, 1995; Fischl, 1988; Leoung, 1990; Slavin, 1992; Schneider, 1992; Hardy 1992; Girad, 1993; Mallolas, 1993; Opravil 1995; Bozzette, 1995; NIH Draft Principles, 1997	Prevent PCP.	9 RCTs support a variety of regimens for patients with CD4 counts < 200, thrush, unexplained fever and/or AIDS defining illnesses. Unexplained fever not included due to potential feasibility problems. Experts recommend lifetime secondary prophylaxis.

2. HIV+ patients who do not have active TB and who have not previously received TB prophylaxis should be offered TB prophylaxis[2] within one month of meeting any of following conditions:
  a. Current PPD > 5 mm;
  b. Provider noting that patient has had PPD > 5 mm administered at anytime since HIV diagnosis;
  c. Contact with person with active TB.
	III	AHCPR, 1994; Hopkins HIV Report, 1997	Prevent development of active TB.	

127

	Indicator	Quality of Evidence	Literature	Benefits	Comments
3.	HIV+ patients who do not have active toxoplasmosis should be offered toxoplasmosis prophylaxis[3] within one month of meeting all of the following conditions: • Toxo IgG positive; • CD4 count dropping below 100; • Completion of therapy for active toxoplasmosis.	I, II	MMWR, 1995; Jacobson 1994; Girad, 1993; Clotet 1991; Clotet, 1992; Bachmeyer, 1994; Richards, 1995	Prevent development of toxoplasmic encephalitis.	RCT evidence for pyramthamine/dapsone treatment of seropositives. Observational and lab evidence for TMP/SMX regimens.
4.	Toxoplasmosis serology should be offered within one month of initial diagnosis of HIV.	II	NIH Draft Principles, 1997; MMWR, 1995; Oskenhendler, 1994	Prevent symptomatic toxoplasmosis.	Screen for asymptomatic toxoplasmosis.
5.	HIV+ patients should be offered MAC prophylaxis[4] within one month of a CD4 count dropping below 50.	I	MMWR, 1995; Nightingale, 1992 and 1993; Pierce, 1996; Havlir, 1996	Prevent development of MAC bacteremia.	
6.	HIV+ patients should have a documented pneumovax.	II	MMWR, 1995	Prevent pnemococcal pneumonia.	
7.	HIV+ patients with a lowest recorded CD4 count of less than 100 should have had a fundoscopic exam in the past year.	III	AHCPR, 1994	Prevent blindness from CMV retinopathy.	Screen for CMV.
8.	VDRL or RPR should be offered within one month of initial diagnosis of HIV infection unless done in past year.	III	AHCPR, 1994; MMWR, 1988	Prevent syphilitic symptoms.	Screen for asymptomatic syphilis.
9.	Sexually active HIV+ patients should be offered a VDRL/RPR annually.	III	AHCPR, 1994; MMWR, 1988	Prevent syphilitic symptoms.	Screen for asymptomatic syphilis.

128

Indicator	Quality of Evidence	Literature	Benefits	Comments
Diagnosis				
10. The following tests should be obtained within one month of initial diagnosis of HIV infection: a. CBC; b. HIV RNA (viral load); c. CD4.	III III III	AHCPR, 1994; Hopkins HIV Report, 1997; Katzenstein, et al., 1996; Mellors, et al., 1997; O'Brien, et al., 1996; MMWR, 1995; O'Brien, 1996; Jurriaans, 1994; Saksela, 1995; Enger, 1996; Dickover, 1994; McIntosh, 1996; Mofenson, 1997; Shearer, 1997; Stein, 1992	(a) Prevent side effects of antiretroviral therapy. (b & c) Reduce morbidity and mortality from HIV infection.	Pap smear and PPD covered in other chapters. (a) Baseline for side effects of future antiretroviral therapy. (b & c) Staging for antiretroviral therapy.
11. HIV+ patients with CD4 counts > 500 should be offered the following tests within 6 months: a. CD4; b. viral loads.	III	AHCPR, 1994; Katzenstein, et al., 1996; Mellors, et al., 1997; O'Brien, et al., 1996; MMWR, 1995; O'Brien, 1996; Jurriaans, 1994; Saksela, 1995; Enger, 1996; Dickover, 1994; McIntosh, 1996; Mofenson, 1997; Shearer, 1997; Stein, 1992	Reduce morbidity and mortality from HIV infection.	Staging for antiretroviral therapy.

	Indicator	Quality of Evidence	Literature	Benefits	Comments
12.	HIV+ patients with CD4 counts < 500 should be offered the following tests within 3 months: a. CD4; b. viral loads.	II	AHCPR, 1994; Katzenstein, et al., 1996; Mellors, et al., 1997; O'Brien, et al., 1996; MMWR, 1995; O'Brien, 1996; Jurriaans, 1994; Saksela, 1995; Enger, 1996; Dickover, 1994; McIntosh, 1996; Mofenson, 1997; Shearer, 1997; Stein, 1992	Staging for antiretroviral therapy.	
13.	HIV+ patients on antiretroviral therapy should have been offered the following tests within the past 3 months: a. CD4; b. viral load; c. CBC.	III	NIH Draft Guidelines, 1997	(a & b) Reduce morbidity and mortality from HIV infection. (c) Prevent side effects of antiretroviral therapy.	Monitoring effects, side effects of antiretroviral therapy. Baseline for side effects of future antiretroviral therapy. Staging for antiretroviral therapy.
Treatment					
14.	HIV+ patients should receive adequate antiretroviral treatment[5] within one month of any of the following conditions being met: a. CD4 > 500 and viral load >30k; b. CD4 350-500 and viral load >10k; c. CD4 <350; d. Any AIDS-defining condition;[6] e. Thrush.	I-III (see comments)	Carpenter, 1996; NIH Draft Guidelines, 1997; Mellors, 1997; O'Brien, 1996	Reduce opportunistic infections, prolong survival.	RCT evidence of decreasing viral load for all regimens and strong observational evidence associating viral load and clinical endpoints. RCT evidence of decreasing progression to AIDS or mortality for certain NRTIs and protease inhibitors. Experts disagree as to the precise levels of CD4 and viral load for initiating therapy. Indicator comprises areas of agreement.
15.	Protease inhibitors should not be prescribed concurrently with astemizole, terfenadine, rifampin or cisapride.	III	NIH Draft Guidelines, 1997	Prevent adverse drug interactions.	Alternatives to contraindicated drugs to available to patients on PI therapy.
Follow-up					
16.	HIV+ patients should be offered viral load measurement within one month of initiation or change in antiretroviral treatment.	III	NIH Draft Guidelines, 1997	Reduce opportunistic infections. Prolong survival.	Monitors effectiveness of therapy.

[1] PCP prophylaxis: TMP/SMX at least 3x/week, Dapsone 100 mg /day, aerosolized pentamidine 300 mg q month, or any toxo regimen (see below)

[2] TB prophylaxis: INH (either 300 mg/d or 900 mg 2x week) + pyrodoxine x12 months or Rifampin 600 mg/day x 12 months

[3] Toxo prophylaxis: Toxoplasmosis prophylaxis: TMP-SMX 1 SS/d or 1 DS 3 x wk, Dapsone 50 mg/d + pyrimethamine 50 mg/wk + leucovorin 25 mg/wk, Dapsone 200 mg/wk + pyrimethamine 75 mg/wk + leucovorin 25 mg/wk.

[4] MAC prophylaxis: Clarithromycin 500 mg qd or bid, Azithromycin > 1000 mg/wk, Rifabutin 300 mg/d

[5] Adequate antiretroviral regimens include: 2 NRTIs + protease inhibitor, 2 NRTIs + NNRTI, 2 NRTIs alone, ddI alone, d4T alone. NRTIs are nucleoside analogues and include: zidovudine (AZT, ZDV), didanosine (Videx, ddI), zalcitabine (HIVID, ddC), stavudine (Zerit, d4T), and lamuvidine (Epivir, 3TC). Protease inhibitors include: saquinavir (Invirase), ritonovir (Norvir), indinavir (Crixivan) and nelfinavir (Viracept). NNRTIs are nonnucleoside reverse transcriptase inhibitors and include: nevirapin (Viramune) and delavirdien (Rescriptor).

[6] AIDS-defining conditions include: candidasis, coccidiomycosis, cryptosporidiosis, cytomegalovirus (CMV), herpes simplex, histoplasmosis, isosporiasis, listeriosis, tuberculosis, mycobacterium avium intrecelluare, pneumocystis carnii pneumoria, recurrent salmonella septicemia, toxoplasmosis, progressive multifocal leucoencephalopathy, cervical cancer, Kaposi's sarcoma, Burkett's lymphoma, lymphoma - immunoblastic, lymphoma - primary of the brain, non-Hodgkin's lymphoma.

Quality of Evidence Codes

I	Randomized controlled trials
II-1	Nonrandomized controlled trials
II-2	Cohort or case analysis
II-3	Multiple time series
III	Opinions or descriptive studies

7. LUNG CANCER

Jennifer Lynn Reifel, MD

The core references for this chapter include the textbook *Cancer Treatment* (Haskell, 1995), CancerNet PDQ Information for Health Care Professionals on non-small cell and small cell lung cancers (CancerNet, 1996) and recent review articles (Karsell, 1993; Miller et al., 1992; Quint et al., 1995; Pugatch et al., 1995; Bragg, 1989; Non-Small Cell Lung Cancer Collaborative Group; Ihde, 1995). Recent review articles were selected from a MEDLINE search identifying all English language review articles published on lung cancer since 1992. Where the core references cited studies to support individual indicators, these have been included in the references. Whenever possible, these have been supplemented with the results of randomized controlled trials.

IMPORTANCE

Lung cancer is the most frequent cause of cancer mortality in the United States. It is estimated that 177,000 people will be diagnosed with lung cancer in 1996 and 158,700 will die from the disease (Parker, 1996). Tobacco inhalation is a major etiologic factor in the development of lung cancer and believed to be the cause of approximately 90 percent of the deaths from lung cancer. Currently, approximately 25 percent of the adult U.S. population smokes. Smoking cessation will be reviewed in another chapter.

SCREENING

Controlled trials of screening with chest x-ray and sputum cytology have failed to show a reduction in lung cancer mortality even for high-risk individuals (Eddy, 1989). There is consensus among the following organizations that screening for lung cancer is not supported by the current evidence: the American Cancer Society, the American College of Radiology, the National Cancer Institute, the U.S. Preventive Services Task Force, and the Canadian Task Force on the Periodic Health Examination. As such, we do not recommend any indicator for the screening or early detection of lung cancer.

DIAGNOSIS

The most common presenting symptoms of lung cancer are related to the local effects of tumor on the airways producing cough, dyspnea, hemoptysis, or chest pain (Patel and Peters, 1993). Many patients present with symptoms of metastatic disease including bone pain, hepatomegaly, or neurologic sequelae of brain lesions. Up to ten percent of lung cancer patients will have clinical manifestations of ectopic hormone production from the tumor, the most common of these being hypercalcemia from PTH-like factor. Occasionally, an unsuspected lung cancer will be discovered on a chest x-ray obtained for some other reason. While many of these symptoms may lead to a diagnostic work-up which reveals the diagnosis of lung cancer, they are not specific for lung cancer. Therefore, we have not proposed a quality indicator on the work-up of a chronic cough, hemoptysis, or other symptoms that may be worrisome for lung cancer.

Frequently lung cancer will be diagnosed during the evaluation of a mass or a solitary pulmonary nodule picked up incidentally on chest x-ray (Toomes et al., 1983; Khouri, 1987; Goldberg-Kahn et al., 1997; Lillington, 1982; Lillington et al., 1993; Libby et al., 1995). A pulmonary mass is defined as a lesion on chest x-ray with a diameter greater than 3 cm. Because lesions greater than 3 cm are almost always malignant, a pathological diagnosis should always be pursued on any patient with such a radiologic finding. Our recommended quality indicator states that any patient with a mass on chest x-ray greater than 3 cm should have documentation of a pathologic diagnosis in the chart (Indicator 1).

A solitary pulmonary nodule is defined as a coin-like lesion on chest x-ray or other imaging study that measures less than 3 cm in diameter. Forty to 50 percent of solitary pulmonary nodules in the United States are caused by lung cancer. When treated at this stage, lung cancer is highly curable, with reported five year survival rates up to 80 percent. Therefore, a pathologic diagnosis should be obtained in every solitary lung nodule that does not have the following benign characteristics:

1. Size is stable when compared with a chest x-ray or other radiographic image from at least two years previously,
2. Nodule has a benign calcification pattern which includes central, diffuse, speckled, laminar or popcorn calcifications, and

134

3. The density of the nodule on CT scan is greater than 168-200
   Hounsfield units.

We recommend a quality indicator requiring that patients without a prior diagnosis of cancer (except non-melanoma skin cancer) who have a solitary pulmonary nodule on chest x-ray, that does not meet at least one of the numbered characteristics above, have documentation of a pathologic diagnosis in the chart (Indicator 2).

While early studies of sputum cytology reported sensitivities up to 98 percent, this appears to have declined, and more recent evaluations suggest it is only 20 to 50 percent sensitive in the current population of lung cancer patients (Karsell et al., 1993; Lukeman, 1973; Kanhouwa et al., 1976; Gagneten et al., 1976; Goldberg-Kahn et al., 1997; Khouri et al., 1987; Karsellet et al., 1993). However, in patients with cancers that involve the central airways, its sensitivity may be as high as 74 percent (Watanabe et al., 1991). If sputum cytology is not diagnostic, fiberoptic bronchoscopy can allow for visualization and biopsy of endobronchial lesions as well as cytology from bronchial washings (Shure, 1985; Edell, 1989; Cortese et al., 1979; Lukeman, 1973). Tumors too peripheral for bronchoscopy can be biopsied with transthoracic needle aspiration or core biopsy, either under CT or fluoroscopic guidance. The diagnostic yield of this technique is approximately 80 to 90 percent with a sensitivity for malignancy ranging from 64 percent to 97 percent, and specificity greater than 95 percent (Khouri et al., 1987; Berquist et al., 1995; Weisbrod, 1990; Gobien et al., 1983; Pavy et al., 1974; Lalli et al., 1978; Westcott, 1981; Gibney et al., 1981). The diagnosis of lung cancer can also sometimes be made from pleural or pericardial fluid cytology, from fine needle aspiration of an enlarged axillary or supraclavicular lymph node, or a lymph node biopsy at mediastinoscopy. In some patients, none of these techniques will be diagnostic and a thoracotomy may be necessary. However, in patients who have what appears to be unresectable lung cancer on imaging, the risk of mediastinoscopy or thoracotomy may not be warranted to make a diagnosis.

Lung cancer is usually divided into non-small cell and small cell lung cancer, and this distinction is relevant because the treatment and prognosis are different. Therefore, we will address the staging, evaluation and treatment of each separately.

135

TREATMENT

Non-Small Cell Lung Cancer

Non-small lung cancer includes three distinct histological types: adenocarcinoma, squamous cell, and large cell carcinoma (Table 7.1). As surgical resection offers the only hope of cure, the treatment approach depends upon determining whether patients are surgically resectable, generally Stages I and II (Table 7.2). In addition, while some patients may have disease which appears resectable, they may not be able to tolerate a lung resection because of poor pulmonary reserve or other medical illnesses. Only about 20 to 35 percent of patients present with resectable disease (Lince et al., 1971; Overholt et al., 1975).

Table 7.1

Histologic Types Of Lung Cancer

Cellular Classification	Subtypes
Non-Small Cell	
Squamous Cell (also epidermoid)	Spindle cell variant
Adenocarcinoma	Acinar Papillary Bronchoalveolar Solid tumor with mucin
Large Cell	Giant cell Clear cell
Adenosquamous	
Small Cell	Oat cell Intermediate Mixed (small cell with other cell types of lung cancer)

The purpose of staging and preoperative evaluation in non-small cell lung cancer is to determine who has disease which can be cured surgically. Methods available for staging include physical exam, laboratory tests, chest x-ray, CT or MRI of the chest, mediastinoscopy, CT of the abdomen, CT or MRI of the brain, and bone scan (Benfield, 1975; Miller et al., 1992; Quint, 1995; Pugatch, 1995). In addition, the morbidity and mortality of lung resections are not inconsequential and must be carefully weighed when deciding to proceed with surgery. Immediate postoperative mortality is age-related but overall is approximately five to eight percent with pneumonectomy and three to five percent with lobectomy. The assessment of pulmonary reserve with pulmonary function tests and arterial blood gas evaluation, as well as the stratification of cardiac risk with surgery, is performed preoperatively to determine if a patient is an operative candidate. The use of these tests and the evaluation of patients for non-operable disease is driven in large measure by expert opinion, the local availability of diagnostic tests, and individual circumstances.

An absolute contraindication to lung resection is the presence of distant metastases. Frequent sites of metastases include bone, liver, adrenal glands, brain, peripheral lymph nodes, and the thorax, including the contralateral lung, mediastinum, and pericardium. Initial staging and evaluation is usually guided by patient symptoms and directed at identifying any metastatic lesion that would necessarily preclude surgery.

Though no currently available studies are sensitive or specific for identifying lung cancer metastases, many tests, including chest x-ray, liver function tests, CT scans, and bone scan, are routinely utilized to evaluate patients who present with lung cancer (Haskell, 1995). While chest x-ray is not very accurate at identifying metastatic lung cancer in the thorax, it has almost always been obtained in the diagnostic evaluation of lung cancer. Lytic lesions of the bones or nodules in the contralateral chest visible on chest x-ray are generally considered evidence of metastatic disease. Liver function tests are almost always elevated with hepatic involvement of lung cancer; however, they are not very specific. A CT scan of the entire abdomen or the use of upper abdomen cuts obtained with chest CT is recommended by some experts to look for metastases in the liver and adrenal glands, although isolated lesions to the liver or the adrenals are rare (Salvatierra et al., 1990; Sider et al., 1988). In fact, approximately 50 percent of the adrenal masses detected in patients with non-small cell lung cancer are benign (Oliver et al., 1984). CT scan of the brain with intravenous contrast is useful to rule out CNS metastases, although it is probably not indicated in patients who do not have symptoms (Jacobs et al., 1977). Routine bone scan is not indicated in patients without symptoms suggestive of bone metastases (pain) as the sensitivity and specificity of bone scan for predicting metastases is 71 percent and 27 percent compared with 100 percent and 54 percent for clinically assessment alone (Michel et al., 1991; Ramsdell et al., 1978). The value of CT imaging of the abdomen and bone scan in patients without symptoms has not been proven. Compelling evidence exists that routine scans of abdomen, brain, and bone have no useful role in patients who do not have clinical or laboratory evidence of metastases to these sites (Bragg, 1989). While each of these tests may be useful in individual circumstances, we do not recommend any of these as quality indicators for the staging of lung cancer.

In addition to distant metastases, locally advanced disease may preclude resection. In general, tumor metastases to scalene or supraclavicular lymph nodes or contralateral hilar or mediastinal lymph nodes; tumor with invasion of the mediastinum, including the heart, great vessels, trachea, esophagus, or carina; or the presence of a malignant effusion with positive cytology (Stage IIIB) are not considered surgically resectable. The management of patients with Stage IIIA disease, which includes tumor involving the mainstem bronchus but not the carina, tumor associated with atelectasis or obstructive pneumonia but not involving the entire lung, or metastases in the ipsilateral mediastinal and subcarinal lymph nodes, remains controversial. In some cases, patients with Stage IIIA disease may be resectable. In any case, if metastatic disease is not present, further staging evaluations are performed to determine if the patient has Stage I, II, or IIIA lung cancer that is potentially resectable.

Once again, chest x-ray, routinely performed for diagnosis of lung cancer, may be useful in determining the extent of disease in the thorax, although it is not very accurate for the evaluation of the mediastinum. Chest x-ray is 61 to 71 percent accurate in detecting hilar adenopathy and 47 to 60 percent accurate in the mediastinal adenopathy, just slightly better than chance (Swensen et al., 1990).

Chest CT, though heavily relied upon, is only slightly better than chest x-ray in helping to evaluate the extent of disease in the chest (Quint et al., 1995). For identifying chest wall invasion, the reported sensitivity of CT ranges from 38 percent to 87 percent with a specificity of 40 to 90 percent. When trying to differentiate between tumors that are greater or less than two cm from the carina, CT has a sensitivity of 56 percent to 89 percent. It is not as useful at determining if the carina or mediastinal structures are involved, which is a more crucial question (Quint et al., 1995; Wursten et al., 1987; Izbicki, 1992; Glazer et al., 1989; Webb et al., 1991). The positive predictive value of CT scan for assessing mediastinal metastases ranges between 49 and 68 percent with sensitivities of 29 to 95 percent and specificities of 46 to 94 percent (Webb et al., 1991; Izbicki et al., 1992; McLoud et al., 1992; Underwood et al., 1979; Inouye et al., 1986; Daly et al., 1987; Dales et al., 1990). While many experts recommend CT scan of the chest for staging, others do not because of its limited ability to predict resectability and mediastinal involvement. In the few studies of magnetic resonance imaging, it does not appear to be any better than CT in the staging of lung cancer (Webb et al., 1991; Webb et al., 1985; Pandovani et al., 1993). Therefore, we do not include routine chest imaging with plain films, CT, or MRI as a recommended quality indicator for the staging of non-small cell lung cancer.

Mediastinoscopy is believed to be the most accurate way of assessing patients for mediastinal lymph node involvement prior to thoracotomy. However, there is no consensus regarding the indications for mediastinoscopy prior to surgical resection (Pearson, 1986; Fishman et al., 1975; Hutchinson and Mills, 1976). Patients who have negative findings at mediastinoscopy have only an eight percent incidence of unresectability at thoracotomy (Pearson, 1986). Well-differentiated peripheral carcinomas with a normal mediastinum on CT scan tend to have an incidence of positive mediastinal node involvement at mediastinoscopy of less than five percent. Therefore, many experts do not believe that patients who have lesions with these characteristics benefit from mediastinoscopy (Hutchinson et al., 1976). Most experts recommend mediastinoscopy in patients whose radiographic studies show mediastinal abnormalities. Many centers perform mediastinoscopy on all patients with mediastinal lymph nodes greater than 1 cm on CT scan (Haskell, 1995). Transbronchial needle aspiration sampling of mediastinal lymph nodes is sometimes used as an alternative to mediastinoscopy prior to thoracotomy (Schure et al., 1984; Wang, 1983). The decision to proceed immediately to thoracotomy or to obtain more staging information with either mediastinoscopy or transbronchial needle aspiration of mediastinal lymph nodes is a complex one that involves weighing the individual patient's risk from the surgical procedure and the likelihood of mediastinal spread of disease based upon the evidence at hand. We therefore do not recommend including mediastinoscopy or mediastinal lymph node biopsy in a quality indicator.

The preoperative evaluation should also attempt to identify patients who would not tolerate lung resection because of poor pulmonary status as well as patients who are at high risk for cardiothoracic surgery. Pulmonary function testing is performed on all patients prior to surgery. If pulmonary function tests show a one second forced expiratory volume of less than 40 percent of predicted or a maximum ventilatory volume level less than 50 percent of predicted, or if the arterial partial pressure of carbon dioxide on a blood gas is greater than 45 mm Hg, resection is generally contraindicated (Shields, 1982; Pett, 1986; Mountain, 1983). Lung perfusion may be assessed using 99mTc-macroaggregated albumin. If the product of the percentage isotope uptake in the contralateral lung and the forced expiratory volume exceeds 0.8 liter, the patient should be able to tolerate a pneumonectomy (Olsen, 1975; Ryo, 1990). As cardiac complications are responsible for about 20 percent of post-operative deaths, and a history of cardiac disease doubles the risk of major surgical morbidity from nine percent to 18 percent, assessing cardiac risk is an important part of determining if a patient can undergo curative resection for lung cancer (Haskell, 1995). At a minimum, an EKG should be performed as part of the preoperative evaluation of every patient prior to lung resection. However, in patients with an abnormal EKG or symptoms suggestive of coronary artery disease, more extensive cardiac evaluation may be indicated. In addition, intractable congestive heart failure or ventricular arrhythmias, as well as a myocardial infarction within three months, are contraindications to surgery (Mountain, 1983).

As a quality indicator for staging and preoperative evaluation of non-small cell lung cancer, we propose that prior to lung resection, patients should have a pathologic diagnosis of lung cancer or a highly suspicious mass on CT scan, pulmonary function tests, and an EKG (Indicator 3).

Resectable Non-Small Cell Lung Cancer (Stage 0, I, and II)

Surgery is the only potentially curative therapy for non-small cell lung cancer. While surgery has not been evaluated in any kind of a controlled manner, the survival of patients with Stage I and II lung cancer who undergo resection with curative intent is generally much better than that of lung cancer patients generally. This is taken as indirect evidence for the efficacy of surgery. The five year survival for Stage I patients is approximately 60 to 70 percent and Stage II is 40 to 50 percent compared with 15 percent overall (Naruke et al., 1988; Mountain, 1988). The surgical resection of non-small cell lung cancer can be accomplished by pneumonectomy, lobectomy, or a segmental or wedge resection depending on the extent of the tumor and lymph node involvement. Local recurrence appears to be greater for patients treated with a segment or wedge resection. Similarly, several non-randomized trials have shown an increase in the local recurrence rate with wedge or segment resections. A survival advantage was noted for lobectomy in patients with tumors greater than 3 cm, but not for those with tumors smaller than 3 cm (Warren et al., 1994; Martini et al., 1995). The Lung Cancer Study Group has compared lobectomy and limited excision for patients with Stage I non-small cell lung cancer in a randomized controlled trial. While there was a reduction in local recurrence for patients treated with lobectomy, there was no difference in overall survival (Ginsberg, 1995).

Patients who are inoperable but have "resectable" disease may be considered for radiation therapy with curative intent, typically 6,000 cGy delivered to the midplane of the tumor. No randomized controlled trials have compared radiation therapy to surgery or to supportive care. Retrospective studies of patients with early stage lung cancer (Stage I and II) treated with radiation therapy demonstrate two year survival rates of 40 to 56 percent and five year survival rates of 10 to 32 percent, though patients with T1 lesions do somewhat better (Hilton, 1960; Zhang et al., 1989; Haffty et al., 1988; Sandler et al., 1990; Talton et al., 1990; Dosoretz et al., 1992). In a retrospective study of patients 70 years and older who had resectable lesions smaller than 4 cm, but who were medically inoperable or refused surgery, survival at five years following radiotherapy was comparable to historical controls who had undergone surgical resection (Noordijk et al., 1988).

Although many patients treated surgically subsequently develop metastases, trials of adjuvant chemotherapy have not demonstrated a statistically significant benefit to survival (Holmes, 1994; Lad et al., 1988; LeChevalier, 1990). Likewise, while postoperative radiation appears to decrease local recurrences, it had no benefit on survival in a controlled trial (Weisenburger et al., 1986).

Because surgical resection offers the best chance of long-term survival for patients with Stage I and II non-small cell lung cancer, we recommend a quality indicator requiring that all patients with adequate pulmonary reserve, who do not have medical record documentation that they are an "unacceptable risk" for surgery and who do not have another metastatic cancer, be offered lung resection with pneumonectomy, lobectomy, or wedge resection (Indicator 4). Patients who are not offered lung resection surgery should be offered radiation therapy to the chest ($\geq$ 5000 cGy) (Indicator 5).

Stage III Non-Small Cell Lung Cancer

The treatment of patients with Stage IIIA lung cancer remains controversial. Select patients (less than ten percent) may be able to undergo a surgical resection, however, patients with mediastinal lymph node involvement do not do as well as patients with early stage disease (Mountain, 1994; Martini et al., 1987). In several randomized trials of immediate surgery or preoperative radiation therapy followed by surgery, preoperative radiation therapy either had no effect or decreased the resectability rate of lung cancer and was associated with shortened survival (Warram et al., 1975; Shields, 1972). The exception to this is superior sulcus tumors which appear to have improved resectability and patient survival when treated with preoperative radiation therapy (Hilaris et al., 1974; Mallams et al., 1964). The results for postoperative radiation therapy in Stage IIIA lung cancer are comparable to those obtained in patients with Stage II lung cancer. Though a few uncontrolled series suggested an improvement in survival with postoperative radiation, the only randomized controlled trial found that while postoperative radiation therapy decreases the local recurrence rate, it does not appear to benefit survival (Weisenburger et al., 1986). Uncontrolled trials and one randomized controlled trial suggest that neoadjuvant chemotherapy with or without radiation therapy may increase the numbers of patients with Stage IIIA lung cancer who are resectable, and may prolong their survival. However, not all the randomized trials comparing this approach to standard therapy have been completed, and the favorable results seen so far may be the result of patient selection (Eagan et al., 1987; Penfield Faber et al., 1989; Weiden et al., 1991; Albain et al., 1991; Rusch et al., 1993; Bitran et al., 1986; Martini et al., 1988; Gralla, 1988; Burkes et al., 1989; Rosell et al., 1994).

For most patients with Stage III lung cancer, the only treatment options are radiation therapy, chemotherapy, or chemotherapy plus radiation therapy. For patients with locally advanced "unresectable" lung cancer, radiation therapy results in only an approximate five percent five year survival rate (Perez et al., 1987; Curran et al., 1990; Cox et al., 1991). Randomized trials comparing radiation therapy alone with radiation therapy and neoadjuvant (up-front), concurrent, or adjuvant (after radiation therapy) chemotherapy have shown that patients with excellent performance status have an improved survival with combined modality therapy when cisplatin was included in the chemotherapy regimen (Trovo et al., 1992; LeChevalier et al., 1991; Mattson et al., 1988; Soresi et al., 1988; Ansari et al., 1991; Morton et al., 1991; Dillman et al., 1990; Schaake-Koning et al., 1992; Sause et al., 1995). A recent meta-analysis of randomized clinical trials showed a ten percent reduction in the risk of death for cisplatin-based chemotherapy with radiation therapy compared with radiation therapy alone (Non-Small Cell Lung Cancer Collaborative Group, 1995).

As a quality indicator for the treatment of patients with Stage III non-small cell lung cancer, we recommend that patients with a good performance status be offered at least one modality of treatment: surgical resection, chemotherapy, or radiation therapy (Indicator 6).

Metastatic Non-Small Cell Lung Cancer (Stage IV)

While chemotherapy is often used in Stage IV non-small cell lung cancer to palliate symptoms and prolong survival, its role in the treatment of patients with metastatic disease remains extremely controversial. Numerous regimens have been tried and none seems superior to the others (Bunn, 1989; Ruckdeschel et al., 1985; Dhingra et al., 1985; Hoffman, 1985; Klatersky et al., 1990; Ruckdeschel et al., 1986; Robert et al., 1984; Einhorn et al., 1986). Randomized trials comparing chemotherapy with no chemotherapy or delayed chemotherapy have produced mixed results. Chemotherapy has been shown in some trials to significantly improve survival from approximately 10 to 17 weeks for control patients to 28 to 37 weeks for patients receiving chemotherapy (Ganz et al., 1989; Rapp et al., 1988; Cartei et al., 1993; Cellerino et al., 1988; Williams et al., 1988; Kaasa et al., 1991). Several meta-analyses of randomized trials of chemotherapy in patients with metastatic non-small cell lung cancer have demonstrated that treatment with chemotherapy is associated with approximately a six week gain in survival compared with patients who receive supportive care (Non-Small Cell Lung Cancer Collaborative Group, 1995). Clinical trials suggest that chemotherapy is most active in patients with good performance status and a pretreatment weight loss of less than ten percent (Gralla, 1989). Although this gain in survival from chemotherapy is minimal, it represents an average of responders and nonresponders. Responders may have a more pronounced survival benefit from chemotherapy. We therefore recommend including a quality indicator which state that patients with metastatic non-small cell lung cancer with a good performance status should be offered chemotherapy (Indicator 7).

Brain Metastases

Brain metastases constitute nearly one third of all recurrences in patients with non-small cell lung cancer, and autopsy data suggest that the incidence may be as high as 50 percent (Van Raemdonck et al., 1992). With symptoms secondary to brain metastases, median survival without therapy is only one month. Whole brain irradiation will effectively palliate symptoms and modestly increase survival by three to six months (Martini, 1986). A solitary brain metastasis may be surgically resected with a marked benefit in long term survival for some individuals. In several series surgical resection of solitary brain lesions has been associated with an increase in median survival from four months to between ten and 16 months (Patchell et al., 1990; Mandell et al., 1986; Van Raemdonck et al., 1992). Patients whose lesions are not surgically resectable may benefit from stereotactic radiosurgery (Alexander et al., 1995; Loeffler et al., 1990). We propose a quality indicator requiring that patients with brain metastases be offered whole brain irradiation, surgical resection, or stereotactic radiosurgery (Indicator 8).

Small Cell Lung Cancer

Untreated, small cell lung cancer is the most aggressive of all types of lung cancer with a median survival of only two to four months. However, it is also the most responsive to chemotherapy and radiation therapy. Chemotherapy results in a four to five-fold improvement in the median survival (CancerNet PDQ, 1996; Haskell, 1995). Because it has such a high propensity for distant metastases, small cell lung cancer is not amenable to surgical treatment (Overholt et al., 1975).

144

Because small cell lung cancer is a systemic disease, and even when not clinically overt metastases are usually present at diagnosis, the TNM staging system is generally not used to stage patients. Instead, a simple system developed by the Veterans Administration Lung Cancer Study group is commonly used. It divides patients into two stages, limited and extensive (Table 7.3). The purpose of the staging in evaluation of small cell lung cancer is to identify patients who have limited disease and that may benefit from radiation therapy to the thorax in addition to systemic chemotherapy. Methods for staging include physical exam, laboratory tests, chest x-ray, CT or MRI of the chest, mediastinoscopy, CT of the abdomen, CT or MRI of the brain, bone scan, and bone marrow biopsy (Miller et al., 1992; Pugatch, 1995). Because there is little consensus on what staging evaluations are appropriate in the absence of specific symptoms, we do not recommend a quality indicator for the staging of small cell lung cancer.

Limited Disease

At the time of diagnosis, approximately one-third of patients will have tumor confined to one hemithorax or the mediastinum or supraclavicular lymph nodes. They are classified as having limited disease. Chemotherapy is the mainstay of treatment for small cell lung cancer; however, randomized controlled trials of combined modality therapy with radiation therapy and chemotherapy have shown a modest but significant improvement in survival compared with chemotherapy alone in patients with limited stage disease.

Chemotherapy produces objective responses in about 80 percent of patients with small cell lung cancer and appears to prolong survival approximately five-fold. Between five and ten percent of patients with limited disease may be cured with chemotherapy alone. In addition, while not well documented in the literature, patients experience a dramatic palliation of symptoms with chemotherapy (Ihde, 1994). A number of chemotherapy regimens have been proven effective in small cell lung cancer. Alternating chemotherapy regimens theoretically could decrease the number of resistant cancer clones, and thereby improve patients' response to chemotherapy. A number of randomized trials have compared alternating drug regimens to standard therapy, but these have not proven to be more effective than the combination of Cisplatin and Etoposide (Goodman et al., 1990; Einhorn et al., 1988; Wolf, 1991). Although the optimal duration of treatment has not been clearly defined, randomized trials comparing longer duration of therapy or maintenance therapy to four to eight cycles of chemotherapy every three to four weeks did not demonstrate any difference in overall survival (Giaccone et al., 1993; Spiro et al., 1989; Bleehen, 1989).

While randomized trials have shown a decrease in local recurrence with the addition of radiation therapy to the thorax, the results of combined modality therapy on overall survival have been mixed (Kies, 1987). However, two meta-analyses of the studies have shown a significant improvement in the absolute three year survival of approximately five percent for those receiving chemotherapy and radiation therapy compared with chemotherapy alone (Pignon, 1992; Warde et al., 1992). Concurrent chemotherapy and radiation therapy may produce better long-term survival than sequential combined modality therapy. Patients in a Phase II SWOG study of concurrent chest irradiation with etoposide and cisplatin chemotherapy had a four year survival of 30 percent compared with ten percent among patients in two earlier SWOG trials of sequential chemotherapy and chest radiation (McCracken et al., 1990). These studies suggest that the effective dose of radiation is in the range of 5,000 cGy or more.

We recommend a quality indicator requiring that all patients with limited disease small cell lung cancer be offered combined modality therapy with radiation therapy ($\geq$ 5000 cGy) to the chest and chemotherapy (Indicator 9).

Extensive Disease

Most patients with small cell lung cancer will present with extensive disease. The same combination chemotherapy regimens used in limited-stage disease appear to effectively palliate symptoms and prolong survival in extensive small cell lung cancer,however, long term survivors remain anecdotal (CancerNet, 1996; Haskell, 1995). Adding radiation therapy to chemotherapy in patients with extensive disease does not appear to prolong their survival. We propose a quality indicator requiring that all patients with extensive small cell lung cancer be offered chemotherapy (Indicator 10).

Palliation of Symptoms

Patients may develop a variety of symptoms secondary to small cell lung cancer including but not limited to cachexia, dyspnea, pain, superior vena cava syndrome, focal neurologic deficits, seizures, and paraneoplastic syndromes. While supportive care may ameliorate some of these symptoms, either chemotherapy or radiation therapy can effectively palliate these symptoms in patients with small cell lung cancer (Kristjansen et al., 1988; Kristensen et al., 1992; Dombernowsky et al., 1978; Kane et al., 1976). We propose quality indicators that require patients with bone pain secondary to metastases and those with brain metastases be offered chemotherapy or local radiation therapy if they have not received it previously (Indicators 11 and 12).

Prophylactic Cranial Irradiation

Brain metastases occur with such frequency in patients with small cell lung cancer that some experts advocate prophylactic cranial irradiation. At diagnosis, ten percent of patients have subclinical brain metastases and brain metastases are present in 50 percent of patients at autopsy (Haskell 1995). Up to ten percent of complete responders present with brain metastases as the only site of recurrence (Haskell, 1995). While prophylactic cranial irradiation has been shown to be effective in reducing the frequency of clinically detected brain metastases, in randomized trials it has not improved survival (Pedersen et al., 1988). Its use has been associated with late neurologic complications, so it remains controversial. Therefore, we do not recommend including prophylactic cranial irradiation as a quality indicator.

FOLLOW-UP

Non-Small Cell Lung Cancer

While up to 50 percent of patients with Stage I and II lung cancer will eventually have a recurrence and die from their disease, there have been no studies on the appropriate follow-up of these patients (CancerNet PDQ, 1996). Patients with isolated recurrences may benefit from resection (as in the case of isolated brain metastasis described above) or other palliative treatment with radiation therapy or chemotherapy. However, the routine use of imaging studies to identify patients for such recurrences or for a second primary lung cancer has not been evaluated.

Patients with Stage III and IV lung cancer generally die from complications of the disease and require supportive care to alleviate their symptoms (CancerNet PDQ, 1996). Again, there are no studies evaluating the appropriate medical follow-up of these patients. As such, we do not recommend a quality indicator for the follow-up of patients with non-small cell lung cancer.

Small Cell Lung Cancer

Patients with small cell lung cancer, except for the rare patient with limited disease, generally die within several years of diagnosis and require supportive care to alleviate their symptoms (CancerNet PDQ, 1996). As in the case of non-small cell lung cancer, there are no studies of the appropriate medical follow-up of patients with small cell lung cancer. As such, we do not recommend a quality indicator for the follow-up of patients with non-small cell lung cancer.

Table 7.2

Definition Of Stages Of Non-Small Cell Lung Cancer

Stage	TNM	Definitions Of Stage For Quality Indicators
Stage 0	T1s N0 M0 - carcinoma in situ	Carcinoma ir situ
Stage I	T1 N0 M0 - Tumor < 3.0 cm surrounded by lung or visceral pleura without evidence more proximal than the lobar bronchus (i.e., not in the main bronchus). T2 N0 M0 - Tumor with any of the following features • > 3.0 cm • involving the mainstem bronchus, 2.0 cm or more distal to the carina • associated with atelectasis or obstructive pneumonia that extends to the hilum but does not involve the entire lung	Tumor may involve the mainstem bronchus but must be 2 cm or more from the carina on chest x-ray, CT scan, or at thoracotomy. All lymph nodes biopsied at mediastinoscopy or thoracotomy are negative.
Stage II	T1 N1 M0 - Tumor < 3.0 cm surrounded by lung or visceral pleura without evidence more proximal than the lobar bronchus (i.e., not in the main bronchus) and metastases in the ipsilateral peribronchial or hilar lymph nodes. T2 N1 M0 - Tumor with any of the following features ≥ 3.0 cm involving the mainstem bronchus, 2.0 cm or more distal to the carina associated with atelectasis or obstructive pneumonia that extends to the hilum but does not involve the entire lung and metastases in the ipsilateral peribronchial or hilar lymph nodes.	Tumor may involve the mainstem bronchus but must be 2 cm or more from the carina on chest x-ray, CT scan, or at thoracotomy. All mediastinal lymph nodes biopsied at mediastinoscopy or thoracotomy are negative but ipsilateral peribronchial or hilar lymph nodes are involved with tumor.

Table 7.2
Definition Of Stages Of Non-Small Cell Lung Cancer
(continued)

Stage	TNM	Definitions Of Stage For Quality Indicators
Stage IIIa	T1-2 N2 M0 - Tumor of any size involving the mainstem bronchus, 2.0 cm or more distal to the carina associated with atelectasis or obstructive pneumonia that extends to the hilum but does not involve the entire lung and metastases in the ipsilateral mediastinal or subcarinal lymph nodes. T3 N0-2 M0 - Tumor of any size with direct extension into the chest wall, diaphragm, mediastinal pleura, parietal pericardium, or in the main stem bronchus < 2.0 cm distal to the carina but not involving the carina and any of the following lymph node statuses: • no lymph nodes involved • metastases in the ipsilateral peribronchial or hilar lymph nodes • metastases in the ipsilateral mediastinal or subcarinal lymph nodes	Mediastinal or subcarinal lymph nodes biopsied at mediastinoscopy or thoracotomy are involved with tumor but no contralateral nodes are involved with tumor. or Tumor extends into the chest wall, diaphragm, mediastinal pleura (but not mediastinal organs), or pericardial pleura, or involves the mainstem bronchus less than 2 cm from but not including the carina either on CT scan or at thoracotomy. Ipsilateral lymph nodes may be involved with tumor but no contralateral lymph nodes are involved with tumor.
Stage IIIb	Any T N3 M0 - Tumor of any size or invasion and metastases in contralateral mediastinal or hilar lymph nodes or any scalene or supraclavicular lymph nodes. T4 any N M0 - Tumor of any size that invades any of the following: mediastinum, heart, great vessels, trachea, esophagus, vertebral body, carina; or a malignant effusion with or without lymph nodes involved.	Scalene or supraclavicular lymph nodes are positive for tumor or contralateral mediastinal lymph nodes are involved with tumor.
Stage IV	Any T Any N M1 - distant metastases are present	Distant metastases are present.

Source: CancerNet, 1996

150

Table 7.3

Definition of Stages of Small Cell Lung Cancer

Stage	Definition of Stage	Definitions of Stage for Quality Indicators
Limited stage	Tumor confined to one hemithorax, the mediastinum, and the supraclavicular nodes, which is encompassable within a "tolerable" radiotherapy port.	Tumor is confined to one half of the chest but may involve the mediastinum on the opposite side and both supraclavicular area lymph nodes.
Extensive stage	Extensive stage small cell lung cancer means tumor that is too widespread to be included within the definition of limited stage disease.	Tumor does not meet the definition of limited disease.

Source: CancerNet, 1996

151

REFERENCES

Albain K, Rusch V, Crowley J, Grifin B, et al. 1991. Concurrent cisplatin (DDP,) VP-16, and chest irradiation (RT) followed by surgery for stages IIA and IIIb non-small cell lung cancer (NSCLC): a Southwest Oncology Group (SWOG) Study (#8805). Abstract # 836. *Proceedings of the ASCO* 10: 244.

Alexander E, Moriarty TM, Davis RB, et al. 1995. Stereotactic radiosurgery for the difinitive noninvasive treatment of brain metastases. *Journal of the National Cancer Intitute* 87: 34-40.

Ansari R, Tokars R, Fisher W, Pennington K, Natravadi R, et al. 1991. A phase III study of thoracic irradiation with or without concomitant cispatin in locoregional unresectable non-small cell lung cancer (NSCLC). Abstract #823. *Proceedings of the ASCO* 10: 241.

Benfield JR. 1975. Current and future concepts of lung cancer. *Archives of Internal Medicine* 83: 93-106.

Berquist TH, Bailey PB, Corese DA, and Miller WE. 1980. Transthoracic needle biopsy: accuracy and complications in relation to location and type of lesion. *Mayo Clinic Proceedings* 55: 475-481.

Bitran J, Golomb HM, Hoffman PC, Albain K, Evans R, Little AG, Purl S, and Skosey C. 1986. Protochemotherapy in non-small cell lung carcinoma. An attempt to increase surgical resectability and survival. *Cancer* 57: 44-53.

Bleehen NM, Fayers PM, Girling DJ, et al. 1989. Controlled trial of twelve versus six courses of chemotherapy in the treatment of small-cell lung cancer: report to the Medical Research Council by its Lung Cancer Working Party. *British Journal of Cancer* 59: 584-590.

Bragg DG. 1989. Imaging in primary lung cancer: the roles of detection, staging, and follow-up. *Seminars in Ultrasound, CT and MR* 10: 453-66.

Bunn PA. 1989. The expanding role of Cisplatin in the treatment of non-small cell lung cancer. *Seminars In Oncology* 16 (Suppl 6): 10-21.

Bunn PA. 1989. Review of trials of Carboplatin in lung cancer. *Seminars In Oncology* 16 (Suppl 5): 27-33.

Burkes R, Ginsberg R, Shepherd F, Blackstein M, Goldberg M, et al. 1989. Neo-adjuvant trial with MVP (Mitomycin C + Vindesine + Cisplatin) chemotherapy for stage III (T1-2, N2, M0) unresectable non-small cell lung cancer (NSCLC). Abstract #860. *Proceedings of the ASCO* 8: 221.

CancerNet PDQ Treatment for Health Professionals, and National Cancer Institute. May 1996. *Non-small Cell Lung Cancer*.

Cartei G, Cartei F, Cantone A, Causarano D, et al. 1993. Cisplatin-Cyclophosphamide-Mitomycin combination chemotherapy with supportive care versus supportive care alone for treatment of metastatic non-small cell lung cancer. *Journal of the National Cancer Institute* 85: 794-800.

Cellerino R, Tummarello D, Porfiri E, Guidi F, et al. 1988. Non small cell lung cancer (NCSLC). A prospective randomized trial with alternating chemotherapy CEP/MEC' versus no treatment. *European Journal of Cancer and Clinical Oncology* 24: 1839-1843.

Cortese DA, and McDougall JC. 1979. Biopsy and brushing of peripheral lung cancer with fluoroscopic guidance. *Chest* 75: 141-145.

Cox JD, Azarnia N, Byhardt RW, Shin KH, et al. 1991. A randomized phase I/II trial of hyperfractionated radiation therapy with total doses of 60.0 Gy to 79.2 Gy: possible survival benefit with ≥ 69.6 Gy in favorable patients with Radiation Therapy Oncology Group stage III non-small cell lung carcinoma: report of Radiation Therapy Oncology Group 83-11. *Journal of Clinical Oncology* 8: 1543-1555.

Curran WJ, and Stafford PM. 1990. Lack of apparent difference in outcome between clinically staged IIIA and IIIB non-small cell lung cancer treated with radiation therapy. *Journal of Clinical Oncology* 8: 409-415.

Dales RE, Stark RM, and Raman S. 1990. Computed tomography to stage lung cancer. Approaching a controversy using meta-analysis. *American Review of Repiratory Disease* 141: 1096-1101.

Daly BDT Jr, Faling LF, Bite G, et al. 1987. Mediastinal lymph node evaluation by computed tomography in lung cancer. *Journal of Thoracic and Cardiovascular Surgery* 94: 664-72.

Dhingra HM, Valdivieso M, Carr DT, Chiuten DF, Farha P, et al. 1985. Randomized trial of three combinations of Cisplatin with Vindesine and/or VP-16-213 in the treatment of advanced non-small cell lung cancer. *Journal of Clinical Oncology* 3: 176-183.

Dillman RO, Seagren SL, Propert KJ, et al. 1990. A randomized trial of induction chemotherapy plus high-dose radiation versus radiation alone in stage III non-small cell lung cancer. *New England Journal of Medicine* 323 (14): 940-945.

Dombernowsky P, and Hansen HH. 1978. Combination chemotherapy in the management of superior vena caval obstruction in small-cell anaplastic carcinoma of the lung. *Acta Medicinae Scandinavia* 204: 513.

Dosoretz DE, Katin MJ, Blitzer PH, et al. 1992. Radiation therapy in the management of medically inoperable carcinoma of the lung: results and implications for future treatment strategies. *International Journal of Radiation Oncology, Biology, Physics* 24 (1): 3-9.

Eagan RT, Ruud C, Lee RE, Pairlero PC, and Gail MH. 1987. Pilot study of induction therapy with cyclophosphamide, doxorubicin, and cisplatin (CAP) and chest irradiation prior to thoracotomy in initially inoperable Stage III M0 non-small cell lung cancer. *Cancer Treatment Report* 71: 895-900.

Eddy DM. 1989. Screening for lung cancer. *Archives of Internal Medicine* 111: 232-237.

Edell ES, and Cortese DA. 1989. Bronchoscopic localization and treatment of occult lung cancer. *Chest* 96: 919-921.

Einhorn LH, Crawford J, Birch R, et al. 1988. Cisplatin plus etoposide consolidation following cyclophosphamide, doxorubicin, and vincristine in limited small-cell lung cancer. *Journal of Clinical Oncology* 6 (3): 451-456.

Einhorn LH, Loehrer PJ, Williams SD, Meyers S, et al. 1986. Random prospective study of Vindesine versus Vindesine plus high-dose Cisplatin versus Vindesine plus Cisplatin plus Mitomycin C in advanced non-small cell lung cancer. *Journal of Clinical Oncology* 4: 1037-1043.

Figlin RA, E Carmack Holmes, and AT Turrisi III. 1995. Non-small cell lung cancer. In: *Cancer Treatment*, 4th ed. Editor Haskell CM, Philadelphia, PA: W.B. Saunders Co.

Fishman NH, and Bronstein MH. 1975. Is mediastinoscopy necessary in the evaluation of lung cancer? *Annals of Thoracic Surgery* 20: 678-686.

Gagneten CB, Geller CE, and del Carmen Saenz M. 1976. Diagnosis of bronchogenic carcinoma through the cytologic examination of sputum, with special reference to tumor typing. *Acta Cytologica* 20: 530-536.

Ganz PA, Figlin RA, Haskell CM, Soto N, and Siau J. 1989. Supportive care versus supportive care and combination chemotherapy in metastatic non-small cell lung cancer. *Cancer* 63: 1271-1278.

Giaccone G, Dalesio O, McVie GJ, et al. 1993. Maintenance chemotherapy in small-cell lung cancer: long-term results of a randomized trial. *Journal of Clinical Oncology* 11 (7): 1230-1240.

Gibney RTN, Man GCW, King EG, and leRiche J. 1981. Aspiration biopsy in the diagnosis of pulmonary disease. *Chest* 80: 300-303.

Ginsberg RJ, and Rubinstein LV. 1995. Randomized trial of lobectomy versus limited resection for T1 N0 non-small cell lung cancer. *Annals of Thoracic Surgery* 60 (5): 615-623.

Glazer HS, Kaiser LR, Anderson DJ, et al. 1989. Indeterminate
    mediastinal invasion in bronchogenic carcinoma: CT evaluation.
    Radiology 173: 37-42.

Gobien RP, Bouchard EA, Gobien BS, Valicenti JF, and Vujic I. 1983. Thin
    needle aspiration biopsy of thoracic lesions: impact on hospital
    charges and patterns of patient care. *Radiology* 149: 65-67.

Goldberg-Kahn B, Healy JC, and Bishop JW. 1997. The cost of diagnosis.
    A comparison of four different strategies in the workup of
    solitary radiographic lung lesions. *Chest* 111: 870-876.

Goodman GE, Crowley JJ, Blasko JC, et al. 1990. Treatment of limited
    small-cell lung cancer with etoposide and cisplatin alternating
    with vincristine, doxorubicin, and cyclophosphamide and chest
    radiotherapy: a Southwest Oncology Group study. *Journal of
    Clinical Oncology* 8: 39-47.

Gralla RJ. 1988. Preoperative and adjuvant chemotherapy in non-small
    cell lung cancer. *Seminars In Oncology* 15: 8-12.

Haffty BG, Goldberg NB, Gerstley J, Fischer DB, and Peschel RE. 1988.
    Resutls of radical radiation therapy in clinical stage I,
    technically operable non-small cell lung cancer. *International
    Journal of Radiation Oncology, Biology, Physics* 15: 69-73.

Hilaris BS, Martini N, Luomanen RKJ, Batata M, and Beattie EJ. 1974. The
    value of preoperative radiation therapy in apical cancer of the
    lung. *Surgical Clinics of North America* 54: 831.

Hilton G. 1960. Present position relating to cancer of the lung.
    Results with radiation therapy alone. *Thorax* 15: 17-18.

Hoffman PC. 1985. *Proceedings of the ASCO* 4: 185.

Holmes AC. 1994. Surgical adjuvant therapy for stage II and stage III
    adenocarcinoma and large cell undifferentiated carcinoma. *Chest*
    106 (6 Suppl): 293S-296S.

Hooper RG, Beechler CR, and Johnson MC. 1978. Radioisotope scanning in
    the initial staging of bronchogenic carcinoma. *American Review of
    Respiratory Disease* 118: 279-286.

Hutchinson CM, and Mills NL. 1976. The selection of patients with
    bronchogenic carcinoma for mediastinoscopy. *Journal of Thoracic
    and Cardiovascular Surgery* 71: 768-773.

Ihde CD. 1995. Small cell lung cancer. State-of-the art therapy 1994.
    Chest 107: 243S-248S.

Inouye SK, and Sox HC. 1986. Standard and computed tomography in the
    evaluation of neoplasms of the chest. A comparative efficacy
    assessment. *Archives of Internal Medicine* 105: 906-924.

Izbicki JR, Thetter O, Karg O, et al. 1992. Accuracy of computed tomographic scan and surgical assessment for staging of bronchial carcinoma. *Journal of Thoracic and Cardiovascular Surgery* 104: 413-420.

Jacobs L, Kinkel WR, and Vincent RG. 1977. 'Silent' brain metastases from lung carcinoma determined by computerized tomography. *Archives of Neurology* 34: 690-693.

Kaasa S, Lund E, Thorud E, Hatlevoll R, and Host H. 1991. Symptmatic treatment versus combiantion chemotherapy for patients with extensive non-small cell lung cancer. *Cancer* 67: 2443-2447.

Kane RC, Cohen MH, Broder LE, and Bull MI. 1976. Superior vena caval obstruction due to small-cell anaplastic lung carcinoma. *Journal of the American Medical Association* 235: 1717-1718.

Kanhouwa SB, and Matthews MJ. 1976. Reliability of cytologic typing of lung cancer. *Acta Cytologica* 20: 229-232.

Karsell PR, and McDougall JC. 1993. Diagnostic tests for lung cancer. *Mayo Clinic Procedures* 68: 288-296.

Khouri NF, Meziane MA, Zerhouni EA, Fishman EK, and Siegelman SS. 1987. The solitary pulmonary nodule. Assessment, diagnosis, and management. *Chest* 91: 128-133.

Khouri NF, Stitik FP, Erozan YS, Gupta PK, Kim WS, Scott WW Jr, et al. 1985. Transthoracic needle aspiration biopsy of benign and malignant lung lesions. *American Journal of Radiology American Journal of Roentgenologyol* 144: 281-288.

Kies MS, Mira JG, Crowley JJ, et al. 1987. Multimodal therapy for limited small-cell lung cancer: a randomized study of induction combination chemotherapy with or without thoracic radiation in complete responders; and with wide-field versus reduced field radiation in partial responders: a Southwest Oncology Group study. *Journal of Clinical Oncology* 4: 592-600.

Klatersky J, Sculier JP, Lacroix G, Dabouis G, Bureau G, et al. 1990. A randomized study comparing Cisplatin or Carboplatin with Etoposide in patients with advanced non-small cell lung cancer: European Organization for Research and Treatment of Cancer Protocol 07861. *Journal of Clinical Oncology* 8: 1556-1562.

Kristensen CA, Kristjansen PEG, and Hansen HH. 1992. Systemic chemotherapy of brain metastases from small cell lung cancer: a review. *Journal of Clinical Oncology* 10: 1498-1502.

Kristjansen PEG, and Hansen HH. 1988. Brain metastases from small cell lung cancer treated with combination chemotherapy. *European Journal of Clinical Oncology* 24: 545-549.

Lad T, Rubeinstein L, and Sadeghi A. 1988. The benefit of adjuvant treatment for resected locally advanced non-small cell lung cancer. *Journal of Clinical Oncology* 6 (1): 9-17.

Lalli AF, McCormack LJ, Zeich M, et al. 1978. Aspiration biopsies of chest lesions. *Radiology* 127: 35-40.

LeChevalier TL, Arriagada R, Quoix E, Ruffie P, Martin M, et al. 1991. Radiotherapy alone versus combined chemotherapy and radiotherapy in nonresectable non-small cell lung cancer: first analysis of a randomized trial in 353 patients. *Journal of the National Cancer Institute* 83: 417-423.

LeChevalier T, Arriagada R, Tarayre M, Lacombe-Terrier M-J, et al. Significant effect of adjuvant chemotherapy on survival in locally advanced non-small cell lung carcinoma. *Journal of the National Cancer Institute* 58:

Libby DM, Henschke CI, and Yandelevitz DF. 1995. The solitary pulmonary nodule: update 1995. *American Journal of Medicine* 99: 491-496.

Lillington GA. 1982. Pulmonary nodules: solitary and multiple. *Clinics in Chest Medicine* 3: 361-367.

Lillington GA, and Caskey CI. 1993. Evaluation and management of solitary and multiple pulmonary nodules. *Clinics in Chest Medicine* 14: 111-119.

Lince L, and Lulu DJ. 1971. Carcinoma of the lung. A comparative series of 687 cases. *Archives of Surgery* 102: 103-107.

Loeffler JS, Kooy HM, Wen PY, et al. 1990. The treatment of recurrent brain metastases with stereotactic radiosurgery. *Journal of Clinical Oncology* 8: 576-582.

Lukeman JM. 1973. Reliability of cytologic diagnosis in cancer of the lung. *Cancer Chemotherapy Reports* 4 (Part 3): 79-93.

Mallams JT, Paulson DL, Collier RE, and Shaw RR. 1964. Presurgical irradiation in bronchogenic carcinoma, superior sulcus type. *Radiology* 82: 1050-1054.

Mandell L, Hilaris B, Sullivan M, et al. 1986. The treatment of single brain metastasis from non-oat cell lung carcinoma: surgery and radiation versus radiation therapy alone. *Cancer* 58: 641-649.

Martini N. 1986. Rationale for treatment of brain metastasis in non-small cell lung cancer. *Annals of Thoracic Surgery* 42: 357-8.

Martini N, Bains MS, Burt ME, et al. 1995. Incidence of local recurrence and second primary tumors in resected stage I lung cancer. *Journal of Thoracic and Cardiovascular Surgery* 109 (1): 120-129.

Martini N, and Flehinger BJ. 1987. The role of surgery in N2 lung cancer. *Surgical Clinics of North America* 67: 1037-1049.

Martini N, Kris MG, Gralla RJ, Bains MS, McCormack PM, Kaiser LR, Burt ME, and Zaman MB. 1988. The effects of preoperative chemotherapy on the resectability of non-small cell lung carcinoma with mediastinal lymph node metastases (N2M0). *Annals of Thoracic Surgery* 45: 370-379.

Mattson K, Holsti LR, Holsti P, Jakobsson M, et al. 1988. Inoperable non-small cell lung cancer: radiation with or without chemotherapy. *European Journal of Cancer and Clinical Oncology* 24: 477-482.

McCracken JD, Janake LM, Crowley JJ, et al. 1990. Concurrent chemotherapy/radiotherapy for limited small-cell lung carcinoma: a Southwest Oncology Group study. *Journal of Clinical Oncology* 8: 892-898.

McLoud TC, Bourgouin PM, Greenberg RW, Kosiuk JP, Templeton PA, et al. 1992. Bronchogenic carcinoma: analysis of staging in the mediastinum with CT by correlative lymph node mapping and sampling. *Radiology* 182: 319-323.

Michel F, Soler M, Imhof E, et al. 1991. Initial staging of non-small cell lung cancer: value of routine radiography bone scanning. *Thorax* 46: 469-474.

Miller JD, Gorenstein LA, and Patterson GA. 1992. Staging: the key to rational management of lung cancer. *Annals of Thoracic Surgery* 53: 170-8.

Morton RF, Jett JR, McGinnis WL, et al. 1991. Thoracic radiation therapy alone compared with combined chemoradiotherapy for locally unresectable non-small cell lung cancer. *Archives of Internal Medicine* 115 (9): 681-686.

Mountain CF. 1988. Prognostic implications of the international staging system for lung cancer. *Seminars In Oncology* 15: 236-245.

Mountain CF. 1994. Surgery for stage IIIA-N2 non-small cell lung cancer. *Cancer* 73: 2589-98.

Mountain CF. 1983. Therapy of stage I and stage II non-small cell lung cancer. *Seminars In Oncology* 10: 71-80.

Naruke T, Goya T, Tsuchiya R, and Suemasu K. 1988. *Journal of Thoracic and Cardiovascular Surgery* 96: 440-7.

Non-small cell lung cancer collaborative group. 1995. Chemotherapy in non-small cell lung cancer: a meta-analysis using updated data on individual patients from 52 randomized clinical trials. *British Medical Journal* 311: 899-909.

Noordijk EM, Clement EP, Hermans J, et al. 1988. Radiotherapy as an alternative to surgery in elderly patients with resectable lung cancer. *Radiotherapy and Oncology* 13 (2): 83-89.

Oliver TW, Bernadino ME, Miller JE, et al. 1984. Isolated adrenal masses in non-small cell bronchogenic carcinoma. *Radiology* 153: 217-18.

Olsen GN, Block AJ, Swenson EW, Castle JR, and Wynne JW. 1975. Pulmonary function evaluation of the lung resection candidate: a prospective study. *American Review of Repiratory Disease* 111: 379-387.

Overholt RH, Neptune WB, and Ashraf MM. 1975. Primary cancer of the lung. a 42-year experience. *Annals of Thoracic Surgery* 20: 511-519.

Pandovani B, Mouroux J, Seksik L, et al. 1993. Chest wall invasion by bronchogenic carcinoma: evaluation with MR imaging. *Radiology* 187: 33-38.

Parker SL, Tong T, Bolden S, and Wingo PA. 1996. Cancer Statistics, 1996. *CA A Cancer Journal for Clinicians* 46: 5-27.

Patchell RA, Ribbs PA, Walsh JW, et al. 1990. A randomized trial of surgery in the treatment of single metastases to the brain. *New England Journal of Medicine* 322: 494-500.

Patel AM, and Peters SG. 1993. Clinical manifestations of lung cancer. *Mayo Clinical Proceedings* 68: 273-277.

Pavy RD, Antic R, and Begley M. 1974. Percutneous needle biopsy of discrete lung lesions. *Cancer* 34: 2109-2117.

Pearson FG. 1986. Lung cancer. The past twenty years. *Chest* 89 (suppl): 200S-205S.

Pedersen AG, Kristjansen PEG, and Hansen HH. 1988. Prophylactic cranial irradiation and small cell lung cancer. *Cancer Treatment Review* 15: 85-103.

Penfield Faber L, Kittle CF, Warren WH, Bonomi PD, Taylor SG, Reddy S, and Lee M-S. 1989. Preoperative chemotherapy and irradiation for Stage III non-small cell lung cancer. *Annals of Thoracic Surgery* 47: 669-677.

Perez CA, Pajak TF, Rubin P, Simpson JR, et al. 1987. Long-term observations of the patterns of failure in patients with unresectable non-oat cell carcinoma of the lung treated with definitive radiotherapy. Report by the Radiation Therapy Oncology Group. *Cancer* 59: 1874-1881.

Pett SB Jr, Wernly JA, and Akl BF. 1986. Lung cancer -- current concepts and controversies. *Western Journal of Medicine* 145: 52-64.

Pignon JP, Arriagada R, Ihde DC, et al. 1992. A meta-analysis of thoracic radiotherapy for small-cell lung cancer. *New England Journal of Medicine* 327 (23): 1618-1624.

Pugatch RD. 1995. Radiologic evaluation in chest malignancies. *Chest* 107: 294S-297S.

Quint LE, Francis IR, Wahl RL, Gross BH, and Glazer GM. 1995. Pre-operative staging of non-small cell carcinoma of the lung: imaging methods. *American Journal of Radiology* 164: 1349-1359.

Ramsdell JW, Peters RP, Taylor AT, Alazraki NP, et al. 1977. Multiorgan scans for staging lung cancer. *Journal of Thoracic and Cardiovascular Surgery* 73: 653-9.

Rapp E, Pater JL, Willan A, Cormier Y, et al. 1988. Chemotherapy can prolong survival in patients with advanced non-small cell lung cancer -- report of a Canadian multicenter randomized trial. *Journal of Clinical Oncology* 6: 663-641.

Robert F, Omura GA, Birch R, Krauss S, and Oldham R. 1984. Randomized phase III comparison of three doxorubicin-based chemotherapy regimens in advanced non-small cell lung cancer: a southeastern cancer study group trial. *Journal of Clinical Oncology* 2: 391.

Rosell R, Gomez-Codina J, Camps C, Maestre J, et al. 1994. A randomized trial comparing preoperative chemotherapy plus surgery with surgery alone in patients with non-small cell lung cancer. *New England Journal of Medicine* 330: 153-158.

Ruckdeschel JC, Finkelstein DM, Mason B, and Creech. 1985. Chemotherapy for metastatic non-small cell bronchogenic carcinoma: EST 2575, Generation V -- a randomized comparison of four cisplatin-containing regimens. *Journal of Clinical Oncology* 3: 72-79.

Ruckdeschel JC, Finkelstein DM, Ettinger DS, Creech RH, Mason BA, Joss RA, and Vogl S. 1986. A randomized trial of the four most active regimens for metastatic non-small cell lung cancer. *Journal of Clinical Oncology* 4: 14-22.

Rusch VW, Albain KS, Crowley JJ, Rice T, et al. 1993. Surgical resection of stage IIIA and stage IIIB non-small cell lung cancer after concurrent induction chemoradiotherapy. *Journal of Thoracic and Cardiovascular Surgery* 105: 97-106.

Ryo UY. 1990. Prediction of postoperative loss of lung function in patients with malignant lung mass: quantitative regional ventilation-perfusion scanning. *Radiologic Clinics of North Americaerica* 28: 657-663.

Salvatierra A, Baamonde C, Llamas JM, Cruz F, and Lopez-Pujol J. 1990. Extrathoracic staging of bronchogenic carcinoma. *Chest* 97: 1052-1058.

Sandler HM, Curran WJ, and Turrisi III AT. 1990. The influence of tumor size and pre-treatment staging on outcome folloing radiation therapy alone for stage I non-small cell lung cancer. *International Journal of Radiation Oncology, Biology, Physics* 19: 9-13.

Sause WT, Scott, Taylor S, et al. 1995. Radiation Therapy Oncology Group (RTOG) 88-08 and Eastern Cooperative Oncology Group (ECOG) 4588: preliminary results of a phase III trial in regionally advanced, unresectable non-small cell lung cancer. *Journal of the National Cancer Institute* 87 (3): 198-205.

Schaake-Koning C, Van dan Bogaert W, Dalesio O, et al. 1992. Effects of concomitant cisplatin and radiotherapy on inoperable non-small cell lung cancer. *New England Journal of Medicine* 326 (8): 524-530.

Schure D, and Fedullo PF. 1984. The role of transcarinal needle aspiration in the staging of bronchogenic carcinoma. *Chest* 86: 693-696.

Shields TW. 1972. Preoperative radiation therapy in the treatment of bronchial carcinoma. *Cancer* 30: 1388-1394.

Shields TW. 1982. Surgical therapy for carcinoma of the lung. *Clinics in Chest Medicine* 3: 369-387.

Shure D, and Fedullo PF. 1985. Transbronchial needle aspiration in the diagnosis of submucosal and peribronchial bronchogenic carcinoma. *Chest* 88: 49-51.

Sider L, and Horejs D. 1988. Frequency of extrathoracic metastases from bronchogenic carcinoma in patients with normal-sized hilar and mediastinal lymph nodes on CT. *American Journal of Roentgenologyol* 151: 893-895.

Soresi E, Clerici M, Grilli R, Borghini U, Zucali R, et al. 1988. A randomized clinical trial comparing radiation therapy v. radiation therapy plus cis-dichlorodiammine platinum (II) in the treatment of locally advanced non-small cell lung cancer. *Seminars In Oncology* 15 (suppl 7): 20-25.

Spiro SG, Souhami RL, Geddes DM, et al. 1989. Duration of chemotherapy in small cell lung cancer: a Cancer Research Campaign trial. *British Journal of Cancer* 59 (4): 578-583.

Swensen SJ, and Brown LR. 1990. Conventional radiography of the hilum and mediastinum in bronchogenic carcinoma. *Radiologic Clinics of North America* 28: 521-538.

Talton BM, Constable WC, and Kersh CR. 1990. Curative radiotherapy in non-small cell carcinoma of the lung. *International Journal of Radiation Oncology, Biology, Physics* 19: 15-21.

Toomes H, Delphendahl A, Manke HG, and Vogt-Moykopg I. 1983. The coin lesion of the lung. A review of 955 resected coin lesions. *Cancer* 51: 534-537.

Trovo M, Minatel E, Veronesi A, Roncadin M, dePaoli A, Franchin G, et al. 1992. Combined radiotherapy and chemotherapy versus radiotherapy alone in locally advanced epidermoid bronchogenic carcinoma. A randomized study. *International Journal of Radiation Oncology, Biology, Physics* 24: 11.

Underwood GH, Hooper RG, Axelbaum SP, and Goodwin DW. 1979. Computed tomographic scanning of the thorax in the staging of bronchogenic carcinoma. *New England Journal of Medicine* 300: 777.

Van Raemdonck DE, Schneider A, and Ginsberg RJ. 1992. Surgical treatment for higher stage non-small cell lung cancer. *Annals of Thoracic Surgery* 54: 999-1013.

Wang KP, Brower R, Haponik EF, and Siegelman S. 1983. Flexible transbronchial needle aspiration for staging of bronchogenic carcinoma. *Chest* 84: 571-576.

Warde P, and Payne D. 1992. Does thoracic irradiation improve survival and local control in limited-stage small-cell carcinoma of the lung? A meta-analysis. *Journal of Clinical Oncology* 10: 890-895.

Warram J, Mountain C, Barkley HT, Ferguson TB, et al. 1975. Preoperative irradiation of cancer of the lung: final report of a therapeutic trial. *Cancer* 36: 914-925.

Warren WH, and Faber LP. 1994. Segmentectomy versus lobectomy in patients with stage I pulmonary carcinoma. *Journal of Thoracic and Cardiovascular Surgery* 107 (4): 1087-1094.

Watanabe U, Shimzu J, Oda M, Iwa T, et al. 1991. Early hilar lung cancer: its clinical aspect. *Journal of Surgical Oncology* 48: 75-60.

Webb WR, Gatsonis C, Zerhouni EA, et al. 1991. CT and MR imaging in staging non-small cell bronchogenic carcinoma: report of the radiologic diagnostic oncology group. *Radiology* 178: 705-713.

Webb WR, Jensen BG, Sollitto R, de Geer G, McCowin M, et al. 1985. Bronchogenic carcinoma: staging with MR compared with staging with CT and surgery. *Radiology* 156: 117.

Weiden PL, S Piantoadosi, and for the Lung Cancer Study Group. 1991. Preoperative chemotherapy (Cisplatin and Fluorouracil) and radiation therapy in stage III non-small cell lung cancer: a phase II studyof the Lung Cancer Study Group. *Journal of the National Cancer Institute* 83: 226-272.

Weisbrod GL. 28 May 1990. Transthoracic percutaneous lung biopsy. *Radiologic Clinics of North America* 647-655.

Weisenburger TH, Holmes EC, Gail M, et al. 1986. Effect of postoperative mediastinal radiation on completely resected stage II and stage III epidermoid cancer of the lung. *New England Journal of Medicine* 315: 1377-1381.

Westcott JL. 1981. Percutaneous needle aspiration of hilar and mediastinal masses. *Radiology* 141: 323-329.

Williams CJ, Woods R, and Page J. 1988. Chemotherapy for non-small cell lung cancer: a randomized trial of Cisplatin/Vindasine v. No Chemotherapy. *Seminars in Oncology* 15: 58-61.

Wolf M, Prisch M, Drings P, et al. 1991. Cyclic-alternating versus response-oriented chemotherapy in small-cell lung cancer: a German multicenter randomized trial of 321 patients. *Journal of Clinical Oncology* 9: 614-624.

Wursten HU, and Vock P. 1987. Mediastinal infiltration of lung carcinoma (T4N0-1): the positive predictive value of computed tomography. *Thoracic and Cardiovascular Surgery* 35: 355-360.

Zhang HX, Yin WB, Zhang LJ, Yang ZY, et al. 1989. Curative radiotherapy of early operable non-small cell lung cancer. *Radiotherapy and Oncology* 14: 89-94.

RECOMMENDED QUALITY INDICATORS FOR LUNG CANCER

The following apply to men and women age 18 and older.

Indicator	Quality of Evidence	Literature	Benefits	Comments
Diagnosis				
1. Patients without a prior diagnosis of cancer (except non-melanoma skin cancer) with a mass (>= 3 cm) on chest x-ray or CT scan of the chest should have one of the following diagnostic endpoints documented in the chart within 2 months of the radiological study: • Chest CT with multiple nodules; • Sputum cytology diagnostic of cancer (expectorated or bronchoscopic washing); • Cytology report from a fine needle aspiration of the mass; • Pathology report from lymph node biopsy that is diagnostic of cancer; • Pathology report from lung biopsy; or • Operative report indicating surgical resection of the mass.	II-2, III	Benfield, 1975; Berquist et al., 1980; Cortese et al., 1979; Edell, 1989; Gagneten, et al., 1976; Gibney et al., 1981; Gobien 1983; Goldberg-Kahn et al., 1997; Haskell, 1995; Kanhouwa and Matthews, 1976; Karsell and McDougall, 1993; Khouri et al., 1987; Lalli et al., 1978; Libby et al., 1995; Lillington 1982; Lillington and Caskey,1993; Lince and Lulu 1971; Lukeman JM 1973; Miller et al., 1992; Overholt 1975; Pavy, 1974; Pugatch, 1995; Quint, 1995; Shure, 1985; Toomes et al., 1983; Watanabe, et al., 1991; Weisbrod 1990; Westcott 1981	Reduce morbidity and mortality from lung cancer.	Experts regard pulmonary lesions >3 cm as probably malignant and recommend prompt resection if possible. Calcification patterns are not predictive of malignancies for masses > 3 cm.

164

Indicator	Quality of Evidence	Literature	Benefits	Comments
2. Patients without a prior diagnosis of cancer (except non-melanoma skin cancer) with a solitary nodule (< 3 cm) on chest x-ray or CT scan of the chest should have one of the following diagnostic endpoints documented in the chart within 2 months of the radiological study: • Report of chest x-ray or CT scan of the chest from at least 2 years prior to the index study which shows a nodule of the same size in the same location; • Chest x-ray or CT scan report describes the nodule as having central, diffuse, speckled, or laminar calcifications; • Chest CT scan report states that the density of the nodule is > 160 Hounsfield units; • Chest CT with multiple nodules; • Sputum cytology, bronchoscopic washing, or bronchoscopic brushing diagnostic of cancer; • Cytology report from a fine needle aspiration of the mass; • Pathology report from lymph node biopsy that is diagnostic of cancer; • Pathology report from biopsy of nodule; • Operative report indicating surgical resection of the mass.	II-2, III	Berquist, 1980; Cortese et al., 1979; Edell et al., 1989; Gagneten et al., 1976; Gibney, 1981; Gobien ,1983; Goldberg-Kahn, 1997; Haskell 1995; Kanhouwa and Matthews 1976; Karsell and McDougall, 1993; Khouri et al., 1987; Khouri, 1985; Khouri, 1987; Lalli et al., 1978; Libby, 1995; Lillington and Caskey, 1993; Lillington, 1982; Lince and Lulu, 1971; Lukeman, 1973; Overholt et al., 1975; Pavy, 1974; Shure, 1985; Toomes et al., 1983; Watanabe et al., 1991; Weisbrod, 1990; Westcott, 1981	Decrease mortality.	40-50% of solitary lung nodules are caused by lung cancer. CT may find smaller nodules than chest x-ray.

Treatment Indicator	Quality of Evidence	Literature	Benefits	Comments
3. Patients with non-small cell lung cancer should have both of the following not more than 3 months prior to lung resection:			Avoid the risk of thoracotomy in patients who would not tolerate a lung resection (reduce mortality from surgery).	Patients with an FEV1<40% are at high risk for respiratory failure following lung resection. A history of cardiac disease doubles the risk of surgical morbidity.
a. Pulmonary function assessment with either pulmonary function tests (FEV1, maximum ventilatory volume) or a quantitative ventilation scan or a quantitative perfusion scan;	II-2, III	Haskell, 1995; Mountain, 1983; Naruke, 1988		
b. EKG.	II-2, III	Haskell, 1995; Warren, 1994		
4. Patients with Stage I and II non-small cell lung cancer should be offered a lung resection (pneumonectomy, lobectomy, or wedge resection) within 6 weeks of diagnosis[1] unless any of the following are documented:	II-2, III	Haskell, 1995; CancerNet, 1996;. Warren et al., 1995; Ginsberg, 1995; Hilton, 1960; Zhang et al., 1989; Haffty et al., 1988	Provide curative treatment to patients who are of acceptable surgical risk.	With surgical resection , the five year survival is approximately 60-70% for Stage I and 40-50% for Stage II lung cancer compared with 15% overall.
a. another metastatic cancer;	II-1, II-2, III	Haskell, 1995; CancerNet Non-small Cell Lung Cancer 1996; Martini, 1995; Ginsberg, 1995		
b. FEV1<40% on pulmonary function tests;	II-1, II-2, III	Haskell, 1995; Olsen et al., 1975; Ryo, 1990; Mountain, 1983; Naruke, 1988		
c. maximum ventilatory volume <50% on pulmonary function tests;	II-2, III			
d. pCO$_2$> 45 mm Hg on an arterial blood gas;	II-2, III			
e. <=0.8 liter perfusion to contralateral lung by quantitative perfusion scan;	II-2, III			
f. documentation in chart that patient is medically "unacceptable risk" for surgery.	II-2, III			

166

	Indicator	Quality of Evidence	Literature	Benefits	Comments
5.	Patients with Stage I or II non-small cell lung cancer who do not undergo a lung resection should be offered radiation therapy to the chest ($\geq$5000 cGy) within 6 weeks of diagnosis.	II-2, III	Haskell, 1995; CancerNet, 1996; Sandler et al., 1990; Talton, 1990; Dosoretz et al., 1992; Noordijk et al., 1988; Holmes et al., 1994; Lad., 1988; LeChevalier,1994	Provide life-prolonging and potentially curative treatment to patients who are not able to undergo surgery.	In a retrospective study of patients 70 years and older who were medically inoperable or refused surgery, survival at 5 years following radiotherapy was comparable to historical controls that had undergone surgical resection.

167

| 6. Patients with Stage III non-small cell lung cancer with good performance status[2] should be offered at least one of the following within 6 weeks of diagnosis:

• thoracotomy with surgical resection of the tumor;

• radiation therapy to the thorax;

• chemotherapy. | II-1, II-2, III | Albain, 1991; Ansari et al., 1991; Bitran et al., 1991; Bunn et al., 1986; Burkes et al., 1989; CancerNet, 1989; Cox et al., 1996; Curran and Stafford et al., 1990; Dillman et al., 1990; Eagan, 1987; Gralla, 1988; Haskell, 1995; Hilaris, 1974; LeChevalier et al., 1991; Mallams, et al., 1964; Martini et al., 1988; Mattson et al., 1988; Morton et al., 1991; Non-small Cell Lung Cancer Collabor-ative Group 1995; Penfield Faber, et al., 1989; Perez et al., 1987; Rosell et al., 1994; Ruck-deschel et al., 1985; Rusch, et al., 1993; Sause et al., 1995; Schaake-Koning et al., 1992; Shields, 1972,; Soresi et al., 1988; Trovo, 1992; Weiden, 1991; Weisen-burger, 1986 | Provide the option of potentially life-prolonging therapy to patients who may benefit. | Randomized trials comparing radiation therapy alone with radiation therapy and chemotherapy have shown that patients with excellent performance status have an improved survival with combined modality therapy. |

168

	Indicator	Quality of Evidence	Literature	Benefits	Comments
7.	Patients with Stage IV non-small cell lung cancer and good performance status should be offered chemotherapy within 6 weeks of diagnosis.	I, II-2, III	Haskell, 1995; CancerNet, 1996; Dhingra et al., 1985; Hoffman, 1985; Klatersky et al., 1990; Ruckdeschel et al., 1986; Robert et al., 1984; Einhorn et al., 1986; Ganz et al., 1989; Rapp et al., 1988; Cartei et al., 1993; Cellerino et al., 1988, Williams et al., 1988; Kaasa et al., 1991; Cancer Bulletin 1991; Non-small cell lung cancer collaborative group, 1995; Bralla 1989; Van Raemdonck et al., 1992; Martini, 1986	Provide the option of potentially life-prolonging therapy to patients who may benefit.	In a recent meta-analysis, patients with metastatic non-small cell lung cancer who received chemotherapy had approximately a six week gain in survival compared with patients who receive supportive care alone. Although this gain in survival from chemotherapy is minimal, it represents an average of responders and nonresponders. Responders may have a more pronounced benefit from chemotherapy.
8.	Patients with non-small cell lung cancer who have metastases on MRI or CT of the brain should be offered one of the following treatments within 2 weeks of the MRI or CT: • radiation therapy to the brain; • surgical resection of the metastasis; • stereotactic radiosurgery.	II-2, III	Patchell et al., 1990; Mandell, 1986; Van Raemdonck et al., 1992; Alexander et al., 1995; Loeffler et al., 1990; CancerNet Non-small Cell Lung Cancer, 1996; Haskell, 1995	Palliate symptoms and prolong life.	Whole brain irradiation will effectively palliate symptoms and modestly increase survival by 3 to 6 months.

169

	Indicator	Quality of Evidence	Literature	Benefits	Comments
9.	Patients with limited small cell lung cancer[4] should be offered combined modality therapy with radiation therapy (>= 5,000 cGy) and chemotherapy within 6 weeks of diagnosis.	I, II-2, III	CancerNet Non-small Cell Lung Cancer, 1996; Haskell, 1995	Provide life-prolonging and potentially curative treatment as well as palliation of symptoms.	Meta-analyses have shown a significant improvement in the absolute 3 year survival of approximately for those receiving chemotherapy and radiation therapy compared with chemotherapy alone (10% versus 5%).
10.	Patients with extensive small cell lung cancer[5] should be offered chemotherapy within 6 weeks of diagnosis.	I, II-2, III	Einhorn et al., 1988; Wolf et al., 1991; Giaccone et al., 1993; Spiro et al., 1989; Bleehen 1989; Kies, 1987; Pignon et al., 1992	Provide life-prolonging treatment as well as palliation of symptoms.	Chemotherapy palliates symptoms and prolongs survival approximately five-fold in small cell lung cancer.
11.	Patients with small cell lung cancer who have metastases on MRI or CT of the brain should be offered either of the following within 2 weeks of diagnosis of brain metastases (unless they have received both previously): • chemotherapy; • radiation therapy to the brain.	II-2, III	Haskell, 1995; CancerNet,1996; Dombernowsky and Hansen, 1978; Kane et al., 1976	Palliate symptoms.	Chemotherapy and radiation therapy are both effective for the palliation of symptoms caused by small cell lung cancer.
12.	Patients with small cell lung cancer who have bone pain and a corresponding positive radiographic study[3] should be offered either of the following within 3 weeks of presenting with the complaint of pain (unless they have received both previously): • chemotherapy; • radiation therapy to the region.	II-2, III	Haskell, 1995; CancerNet,1996; Dombernowsky and Hansen 1978; Kane et al., 1976	Palliate symptoms.	Chemotherapy and radiation therapy are both effective for the palliation of symptoms caused by small cell lung cancer.

Definitions and Examples

[1] If pathological diagnosis has been obtained, date of diagnosis will be considered to be the date of the first pathology report. If pathological diagnosis was not available prior to definitive surgery, date of diagnosis will be the date of the radiological study that suggested the diagnosis of probable lung cancer.
[2] Good performance status: A patient with good performance status may have symptoms from cancer but is still participating in his/her normal daily activities. This would exclude any patients in a nursing home or any patients spending more than just regular sleeping hours in bed.
[3] Corresponding positive radiographic study: This would include a bone scan with increased uptake in the region of pain or an x-ray, CT scan or MRI scan of the painful area that demonstrates a metastasis.
[4] Limited small cell lung cancer: Tumor is confined to one half of the chest but may involve the mediastinum on the opposite side and both supraclavicular area lymph nodes.

[5] Extensive small cell lung cancer: Tumor is not confined to one-half of the chest and involves more than the mediastinum on the opposite side and both supraclavicular area lymph nodes.

Quality of Evidence Codes
I   Randomized controlled trials
II-1   Nonrandomized controlled trials
II-2   Cohort or case analysis
II-3   Multiple time series
III   Opinions or descriptive studies

171

8. PROSTATE CANCER SCREENING

Jennifer Lynn Reifel, MD

The core references for this chapter include recent review articles about prostate cancer screening as well as the recommendations published by the American Cancer Society, the American Urological Association (AUA), the U.S. Preventive Services Task Force (USPSTF), the Canadian Task Force on the Periodic Health Examination, the American College of Physicians (ACP) and the American Academy of Family Physicians (Garnick, 1993; Garnick, 1996, Kramer et al., 1993, Scardino, 1989, Gohagan et al., 1994; Woolf, 1995; Mattlin et al., 1993; USPSTF, 1996; Canadian Task Force, 1994, ACP, 1997; Coley, 1997). Recent review articles were selected from a MEDLINE search identifying all English language review articles published on prostate cancer screening since 1992. Where the core references cited studies to support individual indicators, these have been included in the references. Whenever possible, these have been supplemented with the results of randomized controlled trials.

Screening for prostate cancer remains extremely controversial and no consensus currently exists among the various physician and health policy organizations on whether screening should be routinely offered (Table 8.1). The American Cancer Society recommends that all men age 50 and older receive prostate cancer screening annually with digital rectal examination and prostatic specific antigen (Mettlin, 1993). At the other extreme, the American College of Physicians recommends against screening with the following strongly worded statement: "Routine PSA measurement without a frank discussion of the issues involved is inappropriate. Patients who elect to be screened either by digital rectal examination or PSA measurement, should provide verbal informed consent." (ACP, 1997) In spite of this lack of consensus, screening for prostate cancer with PSA is rapidly spreading and is expected to dramatically increase the numbers of asymptomatic localized cancers diagnosed in the next few years.

Since screening places a burden upon patients (time, expense, potential complications, and anxiety) as well as upon providers and the health care system, five general conditions should be met for any screening intervention to be worthwhile (Hulka, 1988):

173

1. The disease should represent a substantial public health burden;
2. The asymptomatic, non-metastatic phase should be recognizable;
3. Good screening test or tests should be available (i.e., reasonable sensitivity, specificity, and predictive value; low cost; low risk; and acceptable to the person being screened);
4. The curative potential should be substantially better in early stages compared with advanced stages of disease;
5. Treatment of screen-detected cases should decrease cause-specific mortality rates.

We will examine how screening for prostate cancer performs against these criteria.

IMPORTANCE

Prostate cancer (adenocarcinoma) is now the most common cancer in men. In men 75 and older, prostate cancer and benign prostatic hypertrophy together account for about ten percent of office visits each year (Top 30 Diagnoses, 1996). In 1993, the annual incidence of prostate cancer was estimated to be 165,000. Since the FDA approved the use of PSA testing in association with digital rectal examination for early detection of prostate cancer in August 1994, increasing numbers of tumors are being diagnosed and treated before they are palpable. It is estimated that 317,000 new cases will be diagnosed in 1996 and 41,400 deaths in the United States will occur in that same year (Parker et al., 1996). The lifetime risk of dying of prostate cancer is 3.4 percent for American men (Ries et al., 1994). Thus, prostate cancer does represent a substantial health burden.

SCREENING

Recognizable Asymptomatic Phase

The goal of screening or early detection programs for cancer is to identify the disease early enough in the natural history that treatment can significantly change the outcome. In the case of prostate cancer, early detection is defined as before the disease has spread beyond the confines of the gland itself, as treatment for metastatic disease is merely palliative. This is sometimes referred to as "stage shift." That is, screening results in more cases being identified at an earlier stage of the disease. Without screening, approximately 60 percent of newly diagnosed cases of prostate cancer are Stage III or IV and 40 percent are Stage I or II. However, only about half of the cancers clinically determined to be Stage I or II will be found at surgery to be truly organ-confined (Garnick, 1993). The only screening test that has been demonstrated to possibly be associated with "stage shift" is prostate specific antigen (PSA), with up to twice as many cancers being diagnosed while still localized as compared to no screening. However, the increase in the number of localized cancers detected may simply be a reflection of "lead time bias," when a disease is diagnosed earlier in its natural history given the false impression that survival has been prolonged, or "length time bias," which occurs when screening selectively identifies less aggressive tumors because those are the ones that remain clinically "silent" and are therefore preferentially detected in the asymptomatic state (Kramer, 1993). This is especially important because prostate cancer appears to be largely made up of clinically insignificant tumors with only a few becoming clinically important over the patients' lifetimes. Autopsy studies suggest that 40 percent of men age 50 to 70 and 65 percent of men 70 to 80 have clinically undetected prostate cancer, and, in men over 80, it approaches 100 percent (Baron et al., 1995). It is therefore imperative to have survival data from randomized controlled trials of prostate cancer screening to ensure that screening results in "stage shift" and not just "lead time" or "length time" biases.

Accuracy of Screening Tests

The principal screening tests for prostate cancer are digital rectal examination (DRE), the serum tumor marker prostate specific antigen (PSA) and transrectal ultrasound (TRUS). The gold standard against which these tests are compared is pathologic confirmation using biopsy specimens from the prostate (although biopsy may not be a true gold standard because one study has shown that 25 percent of men with one previously negative biopsy were found on a subsequent biopsy to have cancer) (Keetch et al., 1993). Unfortunately, since biopsies are generally not performed in men who have a normal test, the false negative rate of screening tests for prostate cancer are not known. Therefore, the true sensitivity and specificity of DRE, PSA, and TRUS cannot be determined. More importantly, unlike other cancer screening tests currently in use, such as mammography for breast cancer or Pap smears for cervical cancer, no randomized controlled studies have tested the efficacy of screening for prostate cancer in reducing mortality or morbidity.

Digital Rectal Exam

Until recently, DRE was the only screening test for prostate cancer available. Because it requires little time and no significant additional cost, it has generally been integrated into many physicians' routine periodic physical examinations of middle-aged and older men. However, the sensitivity of DRE is limited with studies reporting sensitivities ranging from 18 to 90 percent in detecting prostate cancer in asymptomatic men, when compared against PSA or TRUS (Kramer et al., 1993; Catalona et al., 1991; Catalona et al., 1994; Chodak et al., 1989; Varenhorst et al., 1993; Babaian et al., 1992). It is important to note that these numbers do not represent the true sensitivity of DRE, as neither PSA or TRUS is a "gold standard" test for the detection of prostate cancer. The positive predictive value of DRE is quite low, reported in the range of four to 30 percent. Seventy to 85 percent of men with an abnormal rectal exam have a prostate biopsy without evidence of malignancy (Vihko et al., 1985; Pedersen et al., 1990; Chodak et al., 1989; Pedersen et al., 1990; Richie et al., 1993; Gustafsson et al., 1992). Interrater reliability is only slighly better than chance, even among urologists (Smith et al., 1995; Varenhorst et al., 1993). In addition, two case-controlled studies have failed to show a mortality benefit from screening for prostate cancer with digital rectal exam (Friedman, 1991; Gerber et al., 1993). Hence, even though it is often a traditional part of the periodic physical examination of older men, there is little evidence to recommend periodic DRE alone as a quality indicator of screening for prostate cancer.

Prostate Specific Antigen

PSA is a serine protease which is produced almost exclusively by prostatic epithelial cells (Oesterling, 1991). PSA levels in the serum are increased in prostate cancer (Stamey, 1987; Labrie, 1996). Case control studies have shown that screening with PSA increases the number of men who are found with localized prostate cancer rather than metastatic disease (Auvinen et al., 1996; Catalona et al., 1993; Mettlin, 1994; Labrie et al., 1996; Epstein et al., 1994).

Using a cut-off of 4 ng/dl, PSA has been reported to have a sensitivity of up to 80 percent when compared with prostate biopsy performed to evaluate an abnormal DRE or TRUS. However, it lacks specificity because false positive results are common in patients with benign prostatic hypertrophy (BPH) and prostatitis (Labrie, 1996; Mettlin, 1994; Catalona, 1994). Among men with BPH, 25 to 46 percent will have elevated PSA values (Oesterling, 1991; Sershon, 1994). PSA values in normal men appear to vary by race and age, though this may simply be a reflection of variations in the size or volume of the normal prostate (Oesterling, 1993; Oesterling et al., 1995; Dalkin et al., 1993; Morgan 1996). New techniques currently under investigation which may improve the accuracy of PSA screening include: using age-adjusted and race-adjusted reference ranges (Moul et al., 1995; El-Galley et al., 1995); measuring the PSA density (the PSA concentration divided by the volume of the gland)(Benson et al., 1992; Epstein et al., 1994); the rate of change in PSA levels over time (Carter et al., 1992); and measuring the ratio of free PSA to that complexed to alpha1-chymotrypsin (since the latter accounts for a larger proportion of the PSA in men with prostate cancer than men with BPH)(Oesterling et al., 1995; Stenman et al., 1991; Auvinen et al., 1996). Currently, there are insufficient data to recommend any of these newer techniques, and they are not yet widely available.

Even the reported positive predictive value of 20 to 35 percent may overestimate the percentage of men with an elevated PSA found to have prostate cancer on biopsy. These estimates are derived from studies that included either patients seen at urology clinics or community volunteers, many of whom had obstructive symptoms and therefore were not truly asymptomatic (Cooner et al., 1990; Catalona et al., 1994; Catalona et al., 1993; Richie et al., 1993; Brawer et al., 1992; Bretton, 1994; Muschenheim et al., 1991; El-Galley et al., 1995). Many men undergo biopsies of their prostate for the evaluation of an elevated serum PSA when they do not have prostate cancer. While the PSA test itself is only a blood test of low risk and acceptable to most patients, a prostate biopsy is much more invasive and associated with more discomfort. Two to 40 percent of men who have biopsies are reported to experience minor, self-limited complications; mostly bleeding and urinary tract infections (Desmond, 1993; Webb, 1993). Therefore, any consideration of widespread screening with PSA must take into account the number of prostate biopsies that will result as well.

Combined PSA and DRE

One way to decrease the number of false positive results in screening for prostate cancer is to use both PSA and DRE and only consider the test abnormal if both tests are abnormal. When the results of *both* PSA and DRE are abnormal, the positive predictive value increases from 27 to 32 percent, to 44 to 49 percent. However, combining the two tests significantly reduces the sensitivity of screening (Catalona, 1994; El-Galley, 1994). In one study, when PSA and DRE were combined the sensitivity dropped from 68 percent with PSA and 41 percent for DRE to only ten percent if both were required to be abnormal. When screening for prostate cancer is recommended, current practice usually includes both DRE and PSA, with a positive result on either being sufficient to proceed with further evaluation. The Office of Technology Assessment has estimated that this strategy would result in prostate biopsies for 15 percent of men screened between the ages 50 to 59, 28 percent for ages 60 to 69, and 40 percent at ages 70 to 79 (OTA, 1995).

Transrectal Ultrasound

TRUS has a reported sensitivity of 30 to 68 percent for detecting prostate cancer in asymptomatic men; this is lower than PSA because TRUS cannot distinguish between benign and malignant nodules (Simak et al., 1993; Carter et al., 1989; Catalona et al., 1991; Catalona et al., 1994). When other screening tests are normal the positive predictive value drops to five to nine percent (Babaian, 1992). In addition to these unfavorable test characteristics, TRUS is uncomfortable and costly.

Effectiveness of Screening

"Is cure possible in those for whom it is necessary, and is cure necessary for those in whom it is possible?" - Willet Whitmore

This quote summarizes the dilemma of treating prostate cancer; approximately two-thirds of patients who present with metastatic cancer will die of their disease within five years, with the other one-third succumbing to some other cause of death first (VACURG, 1967). The only hope is to identify cases of prostate cancer before the disease has become widespread so that patients can be cured. However, while most American experts recommend treating localized prostate cancer with either radical prostatectomy or radiation therapy, evidence that such treatment benefits patients is lacking. The only randomized controlled trial of radical prostatectomy with no treatment failed to demonstrate a survival advantage with radical prostatectomy; however, the reliability of this result is often questioned because of small sample size (Graversen et al., 1990). Several non-randomized studies of expectant management (treatment deferred until disease progression) of patients with localized prostate cancer have demonstrated ten year disease-specific survival rates of approximately 85 percent and ten year overall survival rates of approximately 60 percent. These results were comparable to those obtained with radical prostatectomy and radiation therapy (Woolf, 1995; Mettlin, 1993; ACP, 1997; Hulka, 1988). The only randomized controlled trial comparing radical prostatectomy with radiation therapy used time to first treatment failure as its primary endpoint and showed an advantage for radical prostatectomy, though the study is limited both by its choice of endpoint and a different staging between the study arms (Paulson, et al., 1982; Hanks et al., 1988). At the 1987 NIH Consensus Conference on Prostate Cancer, no consensus regarding treatment was reached and none has been reached since.

Both radical prostatectomy and radiation therapy cause substantial complications which negatively impact patient quality of life. Up to 30 percent of men who undergo radical prostatectomy report the need for pads or clamps for incontinence, and about 60 percent report having no erections after surgery, with up to 90 percent reporting no erections sufficient for intercourse during the past month (Garnick et al., 1993; Catalona et al., 1993; Fowler et al., 1993). In addition, surgery is associated with a 0.5 percent to one percent risk of perioperative death (Garnick, 1993). Radiation therapy is associated with a much lower incidence of incontinence and impotence but does carry about a ten percent risk of bowel dysfunction (Garnick, 1993).

Finally, there is controversy as to whether screening identifies those cancers which will have a negative impact on patients' survival or merely insignificant cancers that would not have manifested themselves during the patients' lifetimes. This possibility is significant in prostate cancer because while one-third of men older than 50 will have prostate cancer discovered incidentally at autopsy, clinically apparent prostate cancer develops in only ten percent of men during their lifetime, and only three percent of men die of prostate cancer (Epstein et al., 1986). There is concern that screening programs may identify the two-thirds of prostate cancers, so-called "indolent cancers", that would have never manifest themselves during the individuals' lifetimes, resulting in substantial impact on quality of life (Kramer et al., 1993).

SUMMARY

With respect to the five critera proposed for a worthwhile cancer screening test, the data on current prostate cancer screening are as follows:

1. Prostate cancer does represent a substantial public health burden.

2. The asymptomatic, non-metastatic phase of prostate cancer is recognizable (though studies must be controlled so that "indolent cancers" are not identified and treated).

3. There is incomplete evidence on the test characteristics of DRE and PSA, though it does appear that their sensitivity, specificity, and positive predictive value are not adequate to consider them "good" screening tests. TRUS is not acceptable as a screening test due to its low positive predictive value and also because of patient discomfort, technical difficulty, and cost. Its role remains in the evaluation of abnormal DRE and PSA tests.

4. Because of a lack of randomized controlled trials, it remains controversial as to whether patients with localized prostate cancer live longer when treated with radical prostatectomy or radiation therapy than if not treated until symptoms develop.

5. As yet, there is no evidence that treatment of prostate cancer cases detected by screening decreases cause-specific mortality rates.

Because there is insufficient evidence that screening with either DRE or PSA or both reduces mortality from prostate cancer, and no consensus exists on the issue among organizations that make screening recommendations (Table 8.1), we do not recommend any quality indicators for prostate cancer screening.

Table 8.1

Organizational Recommendations Regarding Prostate Cancer Screening

Organization	Recommendation
American Cancer Society (Mettlin,1993)	Annual examination for early detection of prostate cancer with DRE and PSA beginning at age 50 (annual DRE to begin at age 40 for rectal cancer screening).
American Urological Association (AUANet, 1992)	Annual DRE and PSA measurement substantially increases the early detection of prostate cancer. These tests are most appropriate for male patients 50 years of age and older and for those 40 or older who are at high risk, including those of African-American descent and those with a family history of prostate cancer. Patients in these age/risk groups should be given information about these tests and should be given the option to participate in screening or early detection programs. PSA testing should continue in a healthy male who has a life expectancy of ten years or more.
U.S. Preventive Services Task Force (UPSTF, 1996)	Routine screening for prostate cancer with digital rectal examinations, serum tumor markers (e.g., PSA) or transrectal ultrasound is not recommended (D Recommendation).
Canadian Task Force on the Periodic Health Examination (CTFPHE,1994)	There is poor evidence to include or exclude the DRE from the periodic health examination for men over 50 years of age (C Recommendation). There is insufficient evidence to include PSA screening in the periodic health examination of men over 50 years of age. Exclusion is recommended on the basis of low p sensitivity, specificity, positive predictive value, and the known risk of adverse effects associated with therapies of unproven effectiveness (D Recommendation). There is also fair evidence to exclude transrectal ultrasound from the periodic health examination of asymptomatic men over 50 years of age (D recommendation).

Table 8.1

(continued)

Organization	Recommendation
American College of Physicians (ACP, 1997)	Rather than screening all men for prostate cancer as a matter of routine, physicians should describe the potential benefits and known harms of screening, diagnosis, and treatment; listen to the patient's concerns; and then individualize the decision to screen. The College strongly recommends that physicians help enroll eligible men in ongoing clinical studies.
American Academy of Family Physicians (AAFP, 1996)	Counsel about the known risk and uncertain benefits of screening for prostate cancer (applies to men age 50 to 65).
National Cancer Institute (CancerNet PDQ, 1997)	There is insufficient evidence to establish whether a decrease in mortality from prostate cancer occurs with screening by digital rectal examination, transrectal ultrasound, or serum markers including PSA.

REFERENCES

American Academy of Family Physicians. Summary of Policy Recommendations for Periodic Health Examination.

American College of Physicians. 1997. Position Paper. Clinical Guideline: Part III. Screening for prostate cancer. *Archives of Internal Medicine* 126: 480-484.

AUANet, Urological Services, and Health Policy Statements. May 1992. *Early Detection of Prostate Cancer.* reaffirmed by the AUA Board of Directors,

Auvinen A, Tammela T, Stenman U-H, Uusi-Erkkilä I, et al. 1996. Screening for prostate cancer using serum prostate-specific antigen: a randomised, population-based pilot study in Finland. *British Journal of Cancer* 74: 568-572.

Babaian R, Mettlin C, Kane R, et al. 1992. The relationship of prostate-specific antigen to digital rectal examination and transrectal ultrasonography. *Cancer* 69: 1195-1200.

Baron E, and Angrist A. Incidence of occult adenocarcinoma of the prostate after fifty years of age. *Archives of Pathology* 787-793.

Benson MC, Whang IS, Pantuck A, Ring K, Kaplan SA, Olsson CA, and Cooner WH. 1992. Prostate specific antigen density: a means of distinguishing benign prostatic hypertrophy and prostate cancer. *Journal of Urology* 147: 815-816.

Brawer MK, Chetner MP, Beatie J, Buchner DM, Vessella RL, and Lange PH. 1992. Screening for prostatic carcinoma with prostate specific antigen. *Journal of Urology* 147: 841-5.

Bretton PR. 1994. Prostate-specific antigen and digital rectal examination in screening for prostate cancer: a community based study. *Southern Medical Journal* 87: 720-3.

Canadian Task Force on Periodic Health Examination. 1994. *The Canadian Guide to Clinical Preventive Health Care.* Canada Communication Group, Ottawa, Ont.

CancerNet PDQ Detection and Prevention. May 1997. *Screening for Prostate Cancer.* National Cancer Institute.

Carter HB, Hamper UM, Sheth S, et al. 1989. Evaluation of transrectal ultrasound in the early detection of prostate cancer. *Journal of Urology* 142: 1008-1010.

Carter HB, Pearson JD, Metter J, Brant LJ, Chan DW, et al. 1992. Longitudinal evaluation of prostate-specific antigen levels in men with and without prostate disease. *Journal of the American Medical Association* 267: 2215-2220.

Catalona WJ, and Basler JW. 1993. Return of erections and urinary continence following nerve sparing radical retropubic prostatectomy. *Journal of Urology* 150 (3): 905-907.

Catalona WJ, Richie JP, Ahmann FR, et al. 1994. Comparison of digital rectal examination and serum prostate specific antigen in the early detection of prostate cancer: results of a multicenter clinical trial of 6,630 men. *Journal of Urology* 151: 1283-1290.

Catalona WJ, Smith DS, Ratliff TL, and Basler JW. 1993. Detection of organ-confined prostate cancer is increased through prostate-specific antigen-based screening. *Journal of the American Medical Association* 270: 948-54.

Catalona WJ, Smith DS, Ratliff TL, et al. 1991. Measurement of prostate-specific antigen in serum as a screening test for prostate cancer. *New England Journal of Medicine* 324: 1156-1161.

Chodak GW, Keler P, and Schoenberg HW. 1989. Assessment of screening for prostate cancer using the digital rectal examination. *Journal of Urology* 141: 1136-1138.

Coley CM, Barry MJ, Fleming C, and Mulley AG. 1997. Early detection of prostate cancer. Part I: Prior probablity and effectiveness of tests. *Archives of Internal Medicine* 126: 394-406.

Cooner WH, Mosley BR, Rutherford CL Jr, et al. 1990. Prostate cancer detection in a clinical urological practice by ultrasonography, digital rectal examination and prostate specific antigen. *Journal of Urology* 143: 1146-52.

Dalkin BL, Ahmann FR, and Kopp JB. 1993. Prostate specific antigen levels in men older than 50 years without clinical evidence of prostatic carcinoma. *Journal of Urology* 150: 1837-1839.

Desmond PM, Clark J, Thompson IM, Zeidman EJ, and and Mueller EJ. 1993. Morbidity with contemporary prostate biopsy. *Journal of Urology* 150: 1425-1426.

El-Galley RES, Petros JA, Sanders WH, Keane TE, Galloway NTM, et al. 1995. Normal range prostate-specific antigen versus age-specific prostate-specific antigen in screening prostate adenocarcinoma. *Urology* 46: 200-204.

Epstein JI, Paul G, Eggleston JC, and Walsh PC. 1986. Prognosis of untreated stage A1 prostatic carcinoma: a study of 94 cases with extended follow-up. *Journal of Urology* 136: 837.

Fowler, et al. 1993. Patient-reported complications and follow-up treatment after radical prostatectomy -- the national Medicare experience: 1988-1990 (updated June 1993). *Urology* 42 (6): 622-629.

Friedman GD, Hiatt RA, Quesenberry CP, and Selby JV. 1991. Case-control study of screening for prostatic cancer by digital rectal examinations. *Lancet* 337: 1526-1529.

Garnick MB. 1993. Prostate cancer: screening, diagnosis, and management. *Archives of Internal Medicine* 118 (10): 804-18.

Garnick MB, and Fair WR. 1996. Prostate cancer: emerging concepts. Part I. *Archives of Internal Medicine* 125: 118-125.

Gerber GS, Thompson IM, Thisted R, and Chodak GW. 1993. Disease-specific survival following routine prostate cancer screening by digital rectal examination. *Journal of the American Medical Association* 269: 61-64.

Gohagan JK, Prorok PC, Kramer BS, and Cornett JE. 1994. Prostate cancer screening in the prostate, lung, colorectal and ovarian cancer screening trial of the National Cancer Institute. *Journal of Urology* 152: 1905-1909.

Graversen PH, Nielsen KT, Gasser TC, Corle DK, and Madsen PO. 1990. Radical prostatectomy versus expectant primary treatment in stages I and II prostatic cancer. A fifteen-year follow-up. *Urology* 36 (6): 493-8.

Gustafsson O, Normin U, Almgard LE, Rdereiksson A, et al. 1992. Diagnostic methods in the detection of prostate cancer: a study of a randomly selected population of 2,400 men. *Journal of Urology* 148: 1827-1831.

Hanks GE. 1988. More on the Uro-Oncology Research Group report of radical surgery vs. radiotherapy for adenocarcinoma of the prostate [letter]. *International Journal of Radiation Oncology, Biology, Physics* 14: 1053-54.

Hulka BS. 1988. Cancer screening. Degrees of proof and practical application. *Cancer* 62 (suppl 8): 1776.

Keetch DW, and Catalona WJ. 1993. Update on serial prostatic biopsies in patients with persistently elevated serum prostate specific antigen levels. (Abstract). *Journal of Urology* 149: 303a.

Kramer BS, Brown ML, Prorak PC, Potosky AL, and Gohagan JK. 1993. Prostate cancer screening: what we know and what we need to know. *Archives of Internal Medicine* 119: 914.

Labrie F, Candas B, Cusan L, Gomez J-L, et al. 1996. Diagnosis of advanced or noncurable prostate cancer can be practically eliminated by prostate-specific antigen. *Urology* 47: 212-217.

Mettlin C, Jones G, Averette H, Gusberg SB, and Murphy GP. 1993. Defining and updating the American Cancer Society guidelines for the cancer-related checkup: prostate and endometrial cancers. *CA Cancer a Journal for Clinicians* 43: 42-46.

Mettlin C, Murphy GP, Lee F, Littrup PJ, Chesley A, et al. 1994. Characteristics of prostate cancer detected in the American Cancer Society-National Prostate Cancer Detection Project. *Journal of Urology* 152: 1737-1740.

Morgan TO, Jacobsen SJ, McCarthy WF, Jacobson DJ, McLeod DG, and Moul JW. 1996. Age-specific reference ranges for prostate-specific antigen in black men. *New England Journal of Medicine* 335 (5): 304-10.

Moul JW, Sesterhenn IA, Connelly RR, Douglas T, et al. 1995. Prostate-specific antigen values at the time of prostate cancer diagnosis in African-American men. *Journal of the American Medical Association* 274: 1277-1281.

Muschenheim F, Omarbasha B, Kardijan PM, and Mondou EN. 1991. Screening for carcinoma of the prostate with prostate specific antigen. *Annals of Clinical and Laboratory Science* 21: 371-380.

Oesterling JE. 1991. Prostate specific antigen: a critical assessment of the most useful tumor marker for adenocarcinoma of the prostate. *Journal of Urology* 145: 907-923.

Oesterling JE, Jacobsen SJ, Klee GG, Pettersson K, Piironen T, Abrahamsson PA, et al. 1995. Free, complexed and total serum prostate specific antigen: the establishment of appropriate reference rages for their concentrations and ratios. *Journal of Urology* 154: 1090-1095.

Oesterling JE, Jacobsen SJ, Chute CG, Guess HA, Girman CJ, Panser LA, and Lieber MM. 1993. Serum prostate-specific antigen in a community-based population of healthy men. *Journal of the American Medical Association* 270: 86-864.

Oesterling JE, Kumamoto Y, Tsukamoto T, Girman CJ, Guess HA, Masumori N, Jacobsen SJ, and Lieber MM. 1995. Serum prostate-specific antigen in a community-based population of health Japanese men: lower values than for similarly aged white men. *British Journal of Urology* 75: 347-353.

Office of Technology Assessment. 1995. *Costs and Effectiveness of Prostate Cancer Screening in the Elderly*. Government Printing Office, Washington, D.C.

Parker SL, Tong T, Bolden S, and Wingo PA. 1996. Cancer statistics, 1996. *CA Cancer a Journal for Clinicians* 46: 5-27.

Paulson D, et al. 1982. Radical surgery versus radiotherapy for adenocarcinoma of the prostate. *Journal of Urology* 128: 502-4.

Pedersen KV, Carlsson P, Varenhorst E, et al. 1990. Screening for carcinoma of the prostate by digital rectal examination in a randomly selected population. *British Medical Journal* 300: 1041-1044.

Richie JP, Catalona WJ, Ahmann FR, Hudson MA, et al. 1993. Effect of patient age on early detection of prostate cancer with serum prostate-specific antigen and digital rectal examination. *Urology* 42: 365-74.

Ries LAS, Miller BA, Hankey BF, Kosary CL, Harras A, and Edwards BK. 1994. National Cancer Institute, Bethesda.MD.

Scardino PT. 1989. Early detection of prostate cancer. *Urologic Clinics of North America* 16: 635-655.

Sershon PD, Barry MJ, and Oesterling JE. 1994. Serum prostate-specific antigen discriminates weakly between men with benign prostatic hypertrophy and patients with organ-confined prostate cancer. *European Urology* 25: 281-287.

Simak R, Eisnemenger M, Hainz A, et al. 1993. Is transrectal ultrasonography needed to rule out prostatic cancer with normal findings at digital rectal examination and normal serum prostate-specific antigen? *European Urology* 24: 474-478.

Smith DS, and Catalona WJ. 1995. Interexaminer variability of digital rectal examination for early detection of prostate cancer. *Urology* 45: 70-4.

Stamey TA, Yang N, Hay AR, McNeal JE, Feiha FS, and Redwine E. 1987. Prostate-specific antigen as a serum marker for adenocarcinoma of the prostate. *New England Journal of Medicine* 909-916.

Stenman U-H, Leinonen J, Alfthan H, Rannikko S, Tuhkanen K, and Alfthan O. 1991. A complex between prostate-specific antigen and a1-antichymotrypsin is the major form of prostate-specific antigen in serum of patients with prostatic cancer: assay of the complex improves clinical sensitivity for cancer. *Cancer Research* 51: 222-226.

Top 30 Diagnoses (ICD-9-CM Codes) for Men Ages 65-74 and Men Ages 75+.

US Preventative Services Task Force. 1996. *Guide to Clinical Preventative Services, 2nd ed.* Baltimore: Williams & Wilkins.

Varenhorst E, Berglun K, Logman O, and Pedersen K. 1993. Inter-observer variation in assessment of the prostate by digital rectal examination. *British Journal of Urology* 72: 173-176.

Veterans Administrative Cooperative Urological Research Group. 1967. Treatment and survival of patients with cancer of the prostate. *Surgery, Gynecology and Obstetrics* 124: 1011-7.

Vihko P, Konturi O, Ervast J, et al. 1985. Screening for carcinoma of the prostate: rectal examination and enzymatic radioimmunologic measurements of serum acid phosphatase compared. *Cancer* 56: 173-177.

Webb JA, Shanmuganathan K, and McLean A. 1993. Complications of ultrasound-guided transperineal prostate biopsy, a prospective study. *British Journal of Urology* 72: 775-7.

Woolf SH. 1995. Screening for prostate cancer with prostate-specific antigen. An examination of the evidence. *New England Journal of Medicine* 333: 1401-1405.

9. PROSTATE CANCER TREATMENT

Jennifer Lynn Reifel, MD

The core references for this chapter include the textbook *Cancer Treatment* (Haskell, 1995), CancerNet PDQ Information for Health Care Professionals (National Cancer Institute, 1996) on prostate cancer and recent review articles. Recent review articles were selected from a MEDLINE search identifying all English language review articles published on prostate cancer since 1992 (Garnick, 1993; Garnick and Fair, 1996a; Garnick and Fair, 1996b; Daneshgari and Crawford, 1993; Gibson, 1993; Perez et al., 1993). Where the core references cited studies to support individual indicators, these have been included in the references. Whenever possible, we have cited the results of randomized controlled trials. However, a dearth of such studies in the literature has necessitated that we rely heavily on case analyses and expert opinion to develop quality indicators.

IMPORTANCE

Prostate cancer (adenocarcinoma) is now the most common cancer in men. In men age 75 and older, prostate cancer and benign prostatic hypertrophy together account for about ten percent of office visits each year. In 1993, the annual incidence of prostate cancer was estimated to be 165,000. Since August 1994, when the FDA approved the use of prostate specific antigen (PSA) testing in association with digital rectal examination for early detection of prostate cancer, increasing numbers of tumors have been diagnosed and treated before they were palpable. As a result, it is estimated that 317,000 new cases will be diagnosed in the United States alone in 1996 (Parker et al., 1996).

The natural history of prostate cancer is highly variable. One-third of men older than 50 will have prostate cancer discovered incidentally at autopsy; however, clinically apparent prostate cancer develops in only ten percent of men during their lifetime (Epstein et al., 1986).

Because of the variability in its virulence, and the lack of controlled trials for its treatment, the management of prostate cancer remains confusing and controversial.

SCREENING

Screening for prostate cancer remains extremely controversial. Our rationale for not developing quality indicators for prostate cancer screening, including PSA and digital rectal exam, are discussed in Chapter 8.

However, in spite of a lack of consensus, screening for prostate cancer with PSA is rapidly increasing and is expected to dramatically increase the numbers of asymptomatic localized cancers diagnosed in the next few years.

DIAGNOSIS

Symptoms of urinary obstruction (urgency, nocturia, frequency of urination, and hesitancy) due to an enlarged prostate are the most common presenting symptoms of prostate cancer. These symptoms also occur with benign prostatic hypertrophy. Other less common presenting symptoms of prostate cancer are new onset impotence and less firm penile erections. If the physical exam in a man with symptoms of urinary obstruction is not suggestive of prostate cancer, often the diagnosis will be made incidentally upon pathological examination of tissue obtained during transurethral resection of the prostate (TURP) performed to relieve obstructive symptoms. The quality indicators for the evaluation of obstructive urinary symptoms is discussed in Volume III of this series (see Chapter 4: Benign Prostatic Hyperplasia).

Occasionally, patients present with complaints related to distant metastases, usually back pain from bony lesions, and rarely cord compression or acute urinary retention. When a work-up for back or other bone pain reveals metastatic lesions in a man, a diagnosis of prostate cancer should be pursued because it is the most treatable of the metastatic adenocarcinomas. Further evaluation should include a digital rectal examination of the prostate and PSA (Indicator 1) (Leonard and Nystrom, 1993).

Staging of a cancer refers to the process of determining the presence or absence of factors in a given patient in order to make predictions about the patient's prognosis and make recommendations for treatment. Factors considered useful for predicting prognosis in prostate cancer include the stage and histologic grade of the tumor, the level of the PSA, as well as the patient's age and comorbid conditions (Montie, 1996). Age and comorbidity are important in treatment decisions in prostate cancer because untreated localized prostate cancer has a prolonged course with ten year disease-specific survival rates of approximately 85 percent and ten year overall survival rates of approximately 60 percent (Johansson et al., 1996; Whitmore, 1990; Adolffson, 1993). Therefore, no treatment may be indicated for patients who are not expected to live longer than ten years from the time of the diagnosis of their localized prostate cancer. For this reason we have limited the quality indicators for the treatment of localized prostate cancer with curative intent to men who are expected to live ten years or longer. We have done this by excluding men over 65, as well as men with known coronary artery disease or a second cancer, except for skin cancer (Indicator 5).

The main purpose for staging evaluations when a diagnosis of prostate cancer has been made is to determine if the disease is localized (and thus potentially curable), regionally advanced (and therefore not amenable to surgery with curative intent), or metastatic (not curable).

Two staging systems exist for prostate cancer: the "conventional" or Jewett system, and the American Joint Committee on Cancer/International Union Against Cancer TNM system (see Table 9.1). Below, we review the evidence for the various modalities that have been used to attempt to evaluate prostate cancer stage. Radical prostatectomy with pelvic lymphadenectomy is generally considered the gold standard against which other staging strategies are compared.

Experts recommend obtaining a serum PSA level as part of a staging evaluation for prostate cancer (Garnick and Fair, 1996; Montie, 1996; Oesterling et al., 1993). PSA correlates well with the pathological stage of the tumor: 70 to 80 percent of men with PSA less than 4 ng/ml have localized prostate cancer, and most men with PSA greater than 50 ng/ml have positive pelvic lymph nodes at surgery. However, 60 percent of men with localized prostate cancer have a PSA between 4 and 50 ng/ml so it is not specific enough to be used alone for staging but can be a useful adjunct to other staging evaluations (Partin and Oesterling, 1994; Oeesterling et al., 1993) (Indicator 2).

Digital rectal exam (DRE) is the primary means of determining if the cancer appears to be organ confined (Stage A or B) or has spread locally beyond the confines of the prostate gland (Stage C). However, the sensitivity of DRE for detecting disease that has spread beyond the prostate is only reported to be 10 to 30 percent (Hricak et al., 1987). While transrectal ultrasound has a greater sensitivity for detecting cancer that has spread beyond the confines of the prostate than DRE (66 percent), its specificity is only 46 percent (Rifkin et al., 1990). CT Scan has been shown to have a comparable sensitivity of 67 percent with a specificity of 60 percent for detecting prostate cancer that has spread locally beyond the prostate (Platt et al., 1987). MRI is only slightly better than CT scan at identifying locally invasive prostate cancer, with a reported sensitivity of 75 percent and reported specificity ranging from 57 percent to 88 percent (Rifkin et al., 1993; Hricak et al., 1987).

Identifying patients who have prostate cancer that has already spread to pelvic lymph nodes (Stage IV/D) is even more problematic than identifying locally invasive prostate cancer (Stage III/C). Neither physical exam nor transrectal ultrasound are useful in evaluating pelvic lymph nodes. The sensitivity of CT scan for identifying pelvic lymph nodes involved with prostate cancer is zero percent (Platt, Bree, and Schwab, 1987). MRI has a sensitivity of only four percent for identifying positive lymph nodes in prostate cancer patients (Rifkin et al., 1990). Because of their poor performance in predicting patients with cancer that has spread beyond the prostate (Stage III/C and Stage IV/D), we do not recommend that DRE, transrectal ultrasonography, CT scan, or MRI be included in a quality indicator for the staging evaluation of prostate cancer.

A radionuclide bone scan is generally performed routinely to rule-out bone metastases (Stage IV/D) prior to initiating treatment in most patients with prostate cancer (Garnick, 1993; McGregor et al., 1978). A study evaluating the relationship of the PSA level to bone scan findings in 852 patients with prostate cancer found that no patients with a PSA less than 8.0 ng/ml had bone scan evidence of metastases. Furthermore, 0.5 percent of patients with a PSA less than 10 ng/ml had a positive bone scan, and 0.8 percent of patients with a PSA less than 20.0 ng/ml had a positive bone scan (Oesterling et al., 1993). In accordance with these data and expert opinion (Garnick and Fair 1996; Montie 1996; McGregor et al., 1978; Oesterling et al., 1993), we recommend two quality indicators for the staging of prostate cancer. First, all patients with a new diagnosis of prostate cancer should have a PSA checked within one month of diagnosis or prior to treatment, whichever comes first (Indicator 2). Second, patients with a new diagnosis of prostate cancer and a PSA greater than 10 ng/ml should have a radionuclide bone scan within one month of diagnosis or prior to treatment (Indicator 3).

TREATMENT

Minimal Disease (Stage 0/A1)

No randomized controlled trials have been performed comparing treatment with no treatment in patients with Stage 0/A1 prostate cancer. In case series, rates of disease progression of 5 to 16 percent have been reported with a mean time to progression of six to nine years. However, the survival of men with Stage 0/A1 prostate cancer is comparable to the expected survival of men of similar ages in the general population (Epstein et al., 1986; Lowe and Listrom, 1988; Roy et al., 1990; Thompson and Zeidman, 1989; Zhang et al., 1991). Because the treatments for localized prostate cancer are associated with significant morbidity and survival does not appear to be affected in Stage 0/A1 disease, our proposed quality indicator requires that no treatment be offered to men age 60 and older with Stage 0/A1 disease (Catalona and Basler, 1993; Fowler et al., 1993)(Indicator 4). Since disease progression increases with time, some experts do recommend treating younger men (under age 60) with Stage 0/A1 disease (Catalona and Basler, 1993; Fowler et al., 1993; Epstein et al., 1986). However, because there is no consensus regarding the management of Stage 0/A1 disease in men younger than 60, we have limited our quality indicator to men 60 and older.

Localized Disease (Stage I & II / A2 & B)

Treatment of localized prostate cancer remains controversial. The greatest hope for curing prostate cancer is with radical prostatectomy or radiation therapy while it is still localized. The only randomized controlled trial of radical prostatectomy with no treatment failed to demonstrate a survival advantage with radical prostatectomy. However, the reliability of this result is often questioned because the sample size was only 142, and only 111 of 142 patients included in the trial were available for analysis (Graverson et al., 1990). Several non-randomized studies of expectant management ("watchful waiting") of patients with localized prostate cancer have demonstrated ten year disease-specific survival rates of approximately 85 percent and ten year overall survival rates of approximately 60 percent.

These results are comparable to those obtained with radical prostatectomy and radiation therapy (Perez et al., 1996; Bagshaw et al., 1993; Johansson et al., 1992; Whitmore, 1990; Adolffson, 1993). The only randomized controlled trial comparing radical prostatectomy with radiation therapy used time to first treatment failure as its primary endpoint and showed an advantage for radical prostatectomy (Paulson et al., 1982). But the study has been criticized because the patients treated with radiation were not surgically staged (Hanks, 1988). At the 1987 NIH Consensus Conference on Prostate Cancer, no consensus regarding treatment was reached, and none has been reached since. Still, most American experts recommend definitive treatment for localized prostate cancer for men with a life-expectancy greater than ten years (Gibbons 1993; Bagshaw et al., 1993; Paulson et al, 1982; Perex et al. 1993; Garnick 1993; National Cancer Institute, 1996).

Radical prostatectomy is usually performed via a retropubic approach and newer surgical techniques allow sparing of the neurovascular bundle in order to decrease the incidence of incontinence and impotence. Usually, a pelvic lymphadenectomy is performed prior to the prostatectomy, and the surgeon only proceeds if the lymph nodes are negative for metastatic disease on frozen section. Post-operative complications include incontinence, urethral stricture, rectal injury, impotence, and the morbidity and mortality associated with general anesthesia and a major surgical procedure (30-day mortality of two percent in one study of 10,600 radical prostatectomies). Reports in the literature of complication rates after radical prostatectomy are quite varied. In one large case study of men undergoing the nerve-sparing radical prostatectomy, significant incontinence occurred in six percent of men, while 35 to 60 percent of men who were sexually potent before surgery became impotent following the procedure (Catalona and Basler, 1993). However, in a national survey of Medicare patients who underwent radical prostatectomy in 1988-1990, over 30 percent of men reported the need for pads or clamps for incontinence, and about 60 percent reported having no erections since surgery, with 90 percent reporting no erections sufficient for intercourse during the month prior to the survey (Fowler et al., 1993).

While radioactive implants are used to treat prostate cancer, the most common technique currently in use today is external beam radiation (Garnick, 1993; Bagshaw et al., 1993; Perex et al., 1993). Using a linear accelerator,

67 to 70 Gy is delivered to the prostatic bed and periprostatic tissues over six to seven weeks, with the pelvic lymph nodes receiving approximately 50 Gy. If radiation therapy is chosen as definitive treatment, lymphadenectomy is usually not performed, resulting in those cases which are clinically Stage I or II/A or B but pathologically Stage III or IV/ C or D not being identified. This creates difficulties when trying to compare the outcomes of clinical trials of patients treated with radiation therapy with those treated with radical prostatectomy. The complications of radiation therapy, though infrequent, include diarrhea, proctitis, cystitis, hematuria, rectal bleeding, anal stricture, urethral stricture, rectal ulcer, bowel obstruction. These complications are usually reversible and rarely become chronic (Bagshaw et al., 1993; Garnick, 1993). Sexual potency is generally preserved in the short-term with radiation therapy, but may diminish over time.

Given the lack of clear evidence in favor of a particular treatment for localized prostate cancer, the variable complication rates after radical prostatectomy and radiation therapy, and the need for patients to have the option of a curative treatment when presenting with cancer at a curative stage, we propose a quality indicator specifying that men under age 65 with Stage II/A2&B should have been offered radical prostatectomy or radiation therapy (Indicator 5).

Locally Advanced Disease (Stage III/C)

The optimal treatment for patients with locally advanced prostate cancer is even less clear than that for localized disease. The results of radical prostatectomy in Stage III/C patients are greatly inferior to the results in localized disease (Gibbons, 1993). As surgical removal of the gland is often difficult in Stage III/C prostate cancer, radiation therapy is generally selected for patients with clinical Stage C prostate cancer. The ten year overall survival with both radical prostatectomy and radiation therapy for Stage III/C prostate cancer is about 35 percent. Neoadjuvant androgen ablation therapy has had some success in "downstaging" patients so that PSA levels become undetectable and the remaining cancer is organ confined in more patients at surgery (Labrie et al., 1994; Fair et al., 1993; Gleave et al., 1996). And while one randomized study of radiation therapy with and without androgen ablation showed an advantage in progression-free survival at five years for the arm that received androgen ablation, to date, neoadjuvant androgen ablation has not been shown to provide an advantage in overall survival (Pilepich et al., 1995). Another treatment option for Stage III/C is early androgen ablation therapy (which will be discussed in the Advanced Disease section); but there is no evidence that it prolongs survival. Still another option is expectant management and treatment when necessary to relieve symptoms.

Given the poor ten year survival with locally advanced disease, many experts would recommend more aggressive treatment in younger men (less than age 60) (Haskell, 1995; National Cancer Institute, 1996; Garnick and Fair, 1996a; Gibbons, 1993; Bagshaw et al., 1993). If pathologic staging confirmed Stage III/C disease, many experts would recommend radical prostatectomy, if technically feasible, or radiation therapy with curative intent.

As there is little consensus on how to treat asymptomatic patients with Stage III/C prostate cancer, we do not recommend a quality indicator for the treatment of this group of patients.

Advanced Disease (Stage IV/D)

The most common symptoms of advanced prostate cancer originate from the urinary tract or from bone metastasis. Historically, more than 50 percent of patients present with bone metastases (prior to the advent of PSA screening) (Huggins and Hodges, 1941). Patients with bone pain, visceral involvement, impending cord compression, obstructive urinary symptoms or hydronephrosis should receive androgen ablation therapy for palliation. Experts also generally recommend treating patients with asymptomatic advanced prostate cancer with androgen ablation therapy; however, the data for this are not conclusive. In randomized controlled trials, androgen ablation therapy appears to slow disease progression in Stage IV/D prostate cancer, and may improve overall survival; however, it is not clear if starting androgen ablation therapy early, while patients are still asymptomatic, has an advantage over waiting until patients develop symptoms.

There are multiple approaches to androgen ablation therapy including orchiectomy alone, monotherapy with an luteinizing hormone-releasing hormone

(LHRH) analogue,[1] monotherapy with non-steroidal antiandrogen therapy,[2] or maximal androgen blockade (either orchiectomy or an LHRH analogue and antiandrogen therapy).

The major side-effects of all androgen ablation treatments include impotence (almost universally), breast tenderness, and hot flashes. In addition, with LHRH analogues, many patients experience a flare of bone pain and other symptoms after initiating treatment. Since 1941, orchiectomy has been considered the standard ablation treatment for advanced prostate cancer; however, it has not been compared to no treatment in a randomized trial, nor has it been shown to prolong survival (Huggins and Hodges, 1941). The only randomized placebo-controlled trial of androgen ablation compared DES with placebo. The VACURG study showed a slowing of disease progression in Stage IV/D patients treated with DES 5 mg/day compared with placebo, but overall survival was worse in the group treated with DES (diethylstilbestrol), largely due to an increase in cardiovascular mortality (Veterans Administration, 1967). As treatment with DES in this study was associated with an increase in cardiovascular complications and cardiac mortality, DES has been largely been replaced by the newer drugs (LHRH analogues and antiandrogens). Randomized controlled trials of bilateral orchiectomy, the LHRH analogue goserelin, and DES have shown them all to be equally effective in terms of slowing disease progression (Peeling, 1989; Vogelzang et al., 1995; Kaisary et al., 1991). However, none of these studies answer the specific question of whether immediate therapy has a survival advantage over deferred therapy with androgen blockade for advanced prostate cancer. A randomized trial is currently in progress to try to answer this question (EORTC protocol 30846, 1986).

---

[1] Chronic administration of LHRH analogues causes an inhibition of luteinizing hormone and follicle stimulating hormone release and subsequently a suppression of testicular testosterone secretion similar to that obtained by surgical castration. The commonly used LHRH analogues in the United States are:
  a. leuprolide (Lupron) 1 mg subcutaneous injection daily or 7.5 mg intramuscular injection monthly or 22.3 mg intamuscular injection every 3 months
  b. goserelin acetate (Zoladex) 3.6 mg depot injection monthly or 10.8 mg depot injection every 3 months.

[2] The antiandrogens block the effect of androgens at the receptor level in the prostatic tissue. The antiandrogens commonly used in the United States include:
  a. flutamide (Eulexin) 250 mg by mouth three times a day
  b. bicalutamide (Casodex) 50 mg by mouth daily
  c. nilutamide (Anandron) 300 mg by mouth daily for the first month of treatment followed by 150 mg by mouth daily thereafter.

Some experts advocate maximal androgen blockade therapy with the addition of an antiandrogen to either orchiectomy or an LHRH analogue alone (Labrie et al., 1993). Maximal androgen blockade is thought to be of benefit because, even in the face of medical or surgical castration, adrenal production of testosterone is able to maintain dihydrotesterone levels in the testes of up to 40 percent of normal. The antiandrogens act on the prostate tissue to counter the effect of dihydrotestosterone at the receptor level. Several randomized controlled trials have shown increased progression free survival of three to six months and a survival benefit of approximately six months in patients treated with maximal androgen blockade as compared with monotherapy with an LHRH analogue or orchiectomy, though it only reached statistical significance in two of the studies (Crawford et al., 1989; Keuppens et al., 1990; Beland, 1990; Navaratil, 1987; Janknegt et al., 1993). A subgroup of patients with good performance status and minimal disease (lymph node involvement only) in the NCI randomized trial comparing leuprolide with and without flutamide had a pronounced survival advantage of 20 months (61 versus 41.5 months) when treated with maximal androgen blockade"(Labrie et al., 1993). However, overall the results overall are mixed, and two meta-analyses of monotherapy with LHRH analogues or castration compared with maximal androgen blockade showed no survival advantage for maximal androgen blockade (Bertagna et al., 1994; Prostate Cancer Trialists' Collaborative Group, 1995). Therefore, our quality indicator does not state a preference for maximal androgen blockade over other methods of androgen ablation.

Monotherapy with an antiandrogen is another approach that has been advocated by some experts because it is associated with fewer side-effects (Soloway and Matzkin, 1993). While breast tenderness often still occurs with the antiandrogens, along with occasional nausea and diarrhea, libido and potency, when present before therapy, are generally maintained. Randomized controlled trials comparing monotherapy with an antiandrogen to standard androgen blockade approaches are lacking. In several small randomized trials, flutamide and cyproterone acetate have produced objective responses equal to or greater than DES; yet, no studies have compared patients' survival with these agents (Pavone-Macaluso et al., 1986; Lund and Rasmussen, 1988). Given the absence of data, monotherapy with antiandrogens cannot be considered a standard therapeutic approach for advanced prostatic cancer; however, individual patient preferences may make it the treatment of choice in specific circumstances.

In summary, since patients with Stage IV/D prostate cancer may have a benefit to both progression free survival and overall survival from treatment with androgen ablation, but the evidence in the literature does not clearly support one treatment over the others, we propose as a quality indicator that all men with Stage IV/D prostate cancer be offered at least one of the androgen ablative therapies -- orchiectomy, LHRH analogues, or antiandrogens (Indicator 6).

The advantages of orchiectomy over medical androgen ablation include better patient compliance and lower cost. The disadvantages are the surgical morbidity, the irreversibility of the hormone ablation (and therefore permanence of the associated side-effects), and the psychological effect on the patient of losing his testes. Because it is important for patients to have a choice of treatments, especially when one of them may be psychologically distressing to the patient and equally efficacious alternatives exist, we have developed a quality indicator to ensure that patients who undergo orchiectomy were given a choice. The proposed indicator requires documentation in the patient's chart that he was offered medical androgen ablation as an alternative therapy (Indicator 7).

Hormone Refractory Prostate Cancer

Prostate cancer that progresses while on androgen ablation therapy is termed hormone refractory prostate cancer. Once this occurs, treatment options are limited. A patient being treated with monotherapy when evidence of progression is noted (be it orchiectomy, LHRH analogues, antiandrogens, or DES), especially if symptoms are present, should be given a trial of the maximal androgen blockade. Even when patients progress on maximal androgen blockade, many physicians continue androgen ablation therapy because susceptible cancer cells may still be affected. Other treatment options that exist for hormone refractory prostate cancer include: stopping the antiandrogen (which occasionally produces disease remission), suppression of adrenal androgen production with high dose ketoconazole or aminoglutethamide, estramustine, suramin, or low dose steroids. If patients are asymptomatic and have hormone refractory prostate cancer, the aforementioned approaches can be tried; however, there is no evidence that they delay progression or prolong survival. Thus, many physicians wait until patients have symptoms before instituting any further treatment. If patients have symptoms from prostate cancer that is hormone refractory, any of the above approaches may be used for palliation as well as for trying to slow disease progression. There is insufficient evidence for us to recommend a quality indicator for the treatment of hormone refractory prostate cancer.

Pain from Bone Metastases

Patients with prostate cancer that has metastasized to the bone often suffer from excruciating pain. A primary focus in the care of patients with metastatic prostate cancer is pain control. It is not uncommon for patients to require substantial narcotic analgesia. While narcotics generally provide pain relief, it is often at a cost to quality of life by inducing somnolence, dysphoria, or constipation. Pain may also be relieved, and narcotic requirements reduced, by treatment with androgen blockade or the other systemic therapies discussed in the hormone refractory prostate cancer section. Palliative radiation therapy directed at sites of bony metastases and strontium-89 have been shown to decrease pain and reduce narcotic analgesia requirements in approximately 80 percent of patients. Quality indicators related to pain management are covered in Chapter 11.

Cord Compression

Spinal cord compression develops in approximately seven percent of men with prostate cancer (Osborn et al., 1995). If a patient with prostate cancer develops new or worsening back pain, or neurologic symptoms, spinal cord compression by tumor should be considered. Back pain is the initial symptom in 75 to 100 percent of patients with cord compression. A normal neurologic exam in a patient with back pain does not rule out spinal cord compression. In a study of patients with known malignancy, back pain, and a normal neurologic exam, 36 percent had spinal epidural metastases on myelogram (Rodichok et al., 1981). Plain films of the spine have a sensitivity of 91 percent and a specificity of 86 percent for predicting epidural metastases (Grant et al., 1994). Bone scan has a sensitivity of 91 percent as well, but a specificity of only 53 percent. The positive predictive value of neurologic exam and plain films together varies between studies. False negative rates for ruling-out cord compression with a normal neurologic exam and normal plain film range between zero and 17 percent (Rodichok et al., 1981). The gold standard for diagnosis of spinal cord compression is CT myelogram, and MRI scanning has been shown to have comparable sensitivity and specificity.

Experts recommend that any patient with underlying prostate cancer who develops new or worsening back pain and either has an abnormal neurological exam or abnormal plain films of the spine or an abnormal bone scan undergo either MRI or CT myelogram to rule-out cord compression (Rodichok et al., 1981). As patients with new or worsening back pain who have a normal neurologic exam with normal plain films or bone scan still may have up to a 17 percent risk of cord compression, experts recommend either proceeding on with a MRI and CT myelogram as well or, alternatively, applying a more sensitive test to rule-out metastatic bone disease, a CT scan of the spine (Rodichok et al., 1981). If the CT scan of the spine does not show bony metastases, then spinal cord compression is unlikely. However, if the CT scan of the spine demonstrates metastases, then MRI or CT myelogram are required to evaluate for cord compression.

We recommend that the quality indicator for the evaluation for spinal cord compression include documentation of a normal CT scan of the spine or performance of an MRI or CT myelogram (Indicator 8). No data exist in the literature regarding the time frame in which these tests should be obtained nor how long their results are still valid should new symptoms develop in the future. The evaluation of cord compression is generally considered an emergency, especially if neurologic deficits are present on exam, because the most significant prognostic variables for recovery of function are the severity of weakness at presentation and the duration of paraplegia before treatment is initiated. Therefore, we have selected 24 hours as a conservative maximum allowed time for obtaining an emergent diagnostic study to rule-out cord compression. Given that the median survival for men with hormone refractory prostate cancer is less than ten months (Garnick, 1993), and 57 to 82 percent of men with prostate cancer who develop cord compression are on hormone therapy (suggesting that they have become hormone refractory)(Lund and Rasmussen, 1988), we have allowed for diagnostic tests for cord compression that were obtained up to three months prior to the presenting complaint to satisfy the indicator requirements.

If the radiologic studies are consistent with cord compression, treatment with a minimum dose of dexamethasone (4 mg IV or PO every six hours) should be instituted immediately, followed by palliative radiation therapy or decompressive laminectomy (Lund and Rasmussen, 1988). Randomized controlled trials of higher doses of dexamethasone have not shown an improvement in neurologic recovery (Lund and Rasmussen, 1988). Experts recommend 72 hours of dexamethasone therapy and then a rapid taper (Lund and Rasmussen, 1988). Several retrospective studies comparing decompressive laminectomy alone with decompressive laminectomy followed by radiation therapy have demonstrated a benefit for the latter (Rodichok et al., 1981). When decompressive laminectomy was compared with radiation therapy alone, no differences in functional outcomes were observed; although, in a series of 22 patients with rapidly progressing neurologic signs, 54 percent of those treated with radiation therapy improved and none of those who underwent surgery improved (Lund and Rasmussen, 1988). In general, radiation therapy is considered first line therapy, though in selected cases, such as spinal instability, decompressive laminectomy may be indicated. The dose of radiation in the treatment of cord compression is not well established. Spinal cord toxicity can occur at doses greater than 4500 cGy. No dose-response relationship has been identified in the treatment of spinal cord compression secondary to prostate cancer, but 3000 to 4000 cGy fractionated over two to four weeks is commonly given. We propose that the quality indicator for the treatment of cord compression in prostate cancer include treatment with a minimum dose of 4 mg dexamethasone orally or intravenously every six hours for at least 72 hours, and either radiation therapy (total dose between 3000 cGy and 4500 cGy) or decompressive laminectomy within 24 hours (Indicator 9 and 10).

FOLLOW-UP

Some experts recommend follow-up with DRE and PSA testing for patients with Stage I to III prostate cancer every three months for one year, and every six months thereafter (Garnick, 1993). In addition, prostate biopsy has been recommended 18 to 24 months after completing radiation therapy or if the findings on DRE change (Garnick, 1993). For patients with Stage IV prostate cancer, experts recommend DRE and PSA testing every three months as well as a bone scan, if clinically indicated (Garnick, 1993). However, these

202

frequencies are based upon the follow-up of patients in clinical trials and may not be applicable in a clinical setting where the need to measure treatment outcome at regular intervals does not exist. To date, no studies have evaluated what constitutes necessary and appropriate follow-up of patients with prostate cancer. In addition, there are no data to suggest that diagnosing recurrence earlier leads to prolonged survival or better quality of life asymptomatic patients. As such, follow-up for prostate cancer should be tailored to a patient's symptoms and needs. Therefore, we do not recommend a quality indicator for the follow-up of patients with prostate cancer.

Table 9.1

Definition of Stages of Prostate Cancer

Stage	TNM	Definitions of Stage for Quality Indicators
Stage 0/A1	T1a N0 M0 G1 - clinically inapparent tumor incidentally found in _5 percent of tissue resected by TURP and well-differentiated.	Patient without clinically evident prostate cancer, with prostate cancer found at TURP in _5 percent of tissue resected with a Gleason sum score _4 or described as well-differentiated.
Stage I/A2 & B0	T1a N0 M0 G2-4 - clinically inapparent tumor incidentally found in >5 percent of tissue resected by TURP and well-differentiated. T1b N0 M0 any G - clinically inapparent tumor incidentally found in >5 percent of tissue resected by TURP. T1c N0 M0 any G - clinically inapparent tumor identified by biopsy (performed for evaluation of elevated PSA).	Patient without clinically evident prostate cancer localized to the prostate either: • found at TURP in >5 percent of tissue; • found at TURP in >5 percent of tissue with a Gleason sum score >4 or described as moderately differentiated, poorly differentiated or undifferentiated; • identified by needle biopsy.
Stage II/B	T2 N0 M0 any G - tumor confined to the prostate.	Patient with prostate cancer confined to the prostate palpable on physical exam.
Stage III/C	T3 N0 M0 any G - tumor extends through the prostatic capsule.	Patient with prostate cancer that extends locally outside the prostate.
Stage IV/D	T4 N0 M0 any G - tumor invades or is fixed to adjacent structures other than seminal vesicles. Any T N1-3 M0 any G - tumor involed pelvic lymph nodes. Any T any N M1 any G - tumor has metastasized to sites beyond the pelvic lymph nodes.	Patient with prostate cancer that: • invades adjacent organs such as the anal sphincter, rectum or bladder or adjacent muscles; • involves pelvic lymph nodes; • involves any other part of the body including but not limited to the bones.

REFERENCES

Adolfsson J, Steineck G, and Whitmore WF Jr. 1993. Recent results of management of palpable clinically localized prostate cancer. *Cancer* 72 (2): 310-22.

Bagshaw MA, Kaplan ID, and Cox RC. 1993. Radiation therapy for localized disease. *Cancer* 71: 939-952.

Beland G, Elhilali M, Fradet Y, Laroche B, Ramsey EW, Trachtenberg J, Venner PM, and Tewari HD. 1990. A controlled trial of castration with and without nilutamide in metastatic prostatic carcinoma. *Cancer* 66: 1074-1079.

Bertagna C, de Gery A, Hucher M, et al. 1994. Efficacy of the combination of nilutamide plus orchidectomy in patients with metastatic prostatic cancer: a meta-analysis of seven randomized double-blind trials (1056 patients). *British Journal of Urology* 73 (4): 396-402.

Catalona WJ, and Basler JW. 1993. Return of erections and urinary continence following nerve sparing radical retropubic prostatectomy. *Journal of Urology* 150 (3): 905-907.

Crawford ED, Eisenberger MA, McLeod DG, et al. 1989. A controlled trial of leuprolide with and without flutamide in prostatic carcinoma. *New England Journal of Medicine* 321: 419-424.

Daneshgari F, and Crawford ED. 1993. Endocrine therapy of advanced carcinoma of the prostate. *Cancer* Suppl 71: 1089-1097.

Epstein JI, Paull G, Eggleston JC, and Walsh PC. 1986. Prognosis of untreated stage A1 prostatic carcinoma: a study of 94 cases with extended follow-up. *Journal of Urology* 136: 837.

Fair W, Aprikian A, Cohen D, Sogani O, and Reuter V. 1993. Use of neoadjuvant androgen deprivation therapy in clinically localized prostate cancer. *Clinical and Investigative Medicine* 16: 516-522.

Fowler, et al. 1993. Patient-reported complications and follow-up treatment after radical prostatectomy -- the national Medicare experience: 1988-1990 (updated June 1993). *Urology* 42 (6): 622-629.

Garnick MB. 1993. Prostate cancer: screening, diagnosis, and management. *Archives of Internal Medicine* 118 (10): 804-18.

Garnick MB, and Fair WR. 1996. Prostate cancer: emerging concepts. Part I. *Archives of Internal Medicine* 125: 118-125.

Garnick MB, and Fair WR. 1996. Prostate cancer: emerging concepts. Part II. *Archives of Internal Medicine* 125: 205-212.

Gibbons RP. 1993. Localized prostate carcinoma. *Cancer* 72: 2865-2872.

Gleave ME, Goldenberg SL, Jones EC, Bruchovsky N, and Sullivan LD. 1996. Biochemical and pathological effects of 8 months of neoadjuvant androgen withdrawal therapy before radical prostatectomy in patients with clinically confined prostate cancer. *Journal of Urology* 155: 213-219.

Grant R, Papadopoulos ST, Sandler HM, and Greenberg HS. 1994. Metastatic epidural spinal cord compression: current concepts and treatment. *Journal of Neuro-Oncology* 19: 19-92.

Graversen PH, Nielsen KT, Gasser TC, Corle DK, and Madsen PO. 1990. Radical prostatectomy versus expectant primary treatment in stages I and II prostatic cancer. A fifteen-year follow-up. *Urology* 36 (6): 493-8.

Hainsworth JD, and Greco FA. 1993. Treatment of patients with cancer of an unknown primary site. *New England Journal of Medicine* 329: 257-263.

Hanks GE. 1988. More on the Uro-Oncology Research Group report of radical surgery vs. radiotherapy for adenocarcinoma of the prostate [letter]. *International Journal of Radiation Oncology, Biology, Physics* 14: 1053-54.

Hanks GE, Krall JM, Pilepick MV, Asbell SO, Perez CA, Rubin P, et al. 1992. Comparison of pathologic and clinical evaluation of lymph nodes in prostate cancer: implications of RTOG data for patient management and trial design and stratification. *International Journal of Radiation Oncology, Biology, Physics* 23: 292.

Hricak H, Dooms GC, Jeffrey RB, Avalione A, Jacobs D, Benton WK, et al. 1987. Prostatic carcinoma: staging by clinical assessment, CT and MR imaging. *Radiology* 162: 331-6.

Huggins C, and Hodges CV. 1941. Studies of prostatic cancer: I. Effect of castration, estrogen, and androgen injections on serum phosphatases in metastatic carcinoma of the prostate. *Cancer Research* 1: 293-297.

Janknegt RA, Abbou CC, and Bartoletti R. 1993. Orchiectomy and Anandron (nilutamide) or placebo as treatment of metastatic prostatic cancer in a multinational double-blind randomized trial. *Journal of Urology* 149: 77-83.

Johansson JE, Adami HO, Andersson SO, Bergstrom R, Homberg L, and Krusemo UB. 1992. High 10-year survival rate in patients with early, untreated prostatic cancer. *Journal of the American Medical Association* 267 (16): 2191-2196.

Kaisary AV, Tyrrell CJ, Peeling WB, et al. 1991. Comparison of LHRH analogue (Zoladex) with orchiectomy in patients with metastatic prostatic carcinoma. *British Journal of Urology* 67 (5): 502-508.

Keuppens F, Denis L, Smith P, Carvalho AP, Newling D, Bond A, Sylvester R, DePauw M, Vermeylen K, Ongena P, and and the EORTC GU Group. 1990. Zoladex and flutamide versus bilateral orchiectomy. A randomized Phase III EORTC 30853 study. *Cancer* 5: 1057.

Labrie F, Belanger A, Simard J, Labrie C, and Dupont A. 1993. Combination therapy for prostate cancer. Endocrine and biologic basis of its choice as new standard first-line therapy. *Cancer* 71: 1059-67.

Labrie F, Cusan L, Gomez J-L, Diamond P, et al. 1994. Down-staging of early stage prostate cancer before radical prostatectomy: the first randomized trial of neoadjuvant combination therapy with flutamide and a luteinizing hormone-releasing agonist. *Urology Symposium* 44: 29-37.

Leonard RJ, and Nystrom JS. 1993. Diagnostic evaluation of patients with carcinoma of unknown primary tumor site. *Seminars in Oncology* 20: 244-250.

Lowe BA, and Listrom MB. 1988. Incidental carcinoma of the prostate: an analysis of the predictors of progression. *Journal of Urology* 140: 1340.

Lund F, and Rasmussen F. 1988. Flutamide versus stilboestrol in the management of advanced prostatic cancer. *British Journal of Urology* 61: 140-2.

McGregor B, Tulloch AGS, Quinlan MF, and Lovegrove F. 1978. The role of bone scanning in the assesment of prostatic carcinoma. *British Journal of Urology* 50: 178-181.

Montie JE. 1996. Current prognostic factors for prostate carcinoma. *Cancer* 78 (2): 341-4.

Navaratil D. 1987. Double blind study of Anandron versus placebo in Stage D2 prostate cancer patients receiving buserelin. In *Prostate cancer: part A: research, endocrine treatment, and histopathology*. editors Murphy G, Khoury S, Kuss R, Chatelan C, and Denis L, 401-410. New York: Alan R. Liss.

Oesterling JE, Martin SK, Berstralh MS, and Lowe FC. 1993. The use of prostate-specific antigen in staging patients with newly diagnosed prostate cancer. *Journal of the American Medical Association* 269: 57-60.

Osborn JL, Getzenberg RH, and Trump D. 1995. Spinal cord compression in prostate cancer. *Journal of Neuro-Oncology* 23: 135-147.

Parker SL, Tong T, Bolden S, and Wingo PA. 1996. Cancer statistics, 1996. *CA Cancer a Journal for Clinicians* 46: 5-27.

Partin AW, and Oesterling JE. 1994. The clinical usefulness of prostate specific antigen: update 1994. *Journal of Urology* 152: 1358-1368.

Paulson DF, et al. 1982. Radical surgery versus radiotherapy for adenocarcinoma of the prostate. *Journal of Urology* 128: 502-4.

Pavone-Macaluso M, De-Voogt HJ, Viggian G, Barasolo E, Lardennois B, de Pauw M, et al. 1986. Comparison of diethylstilbestrol, CPA and medroxyprogesterone acetate in the treatment of advanced prostatic cancer. *Journal of Urology* 136: 624-31.

Peeling WB. 1989. Phase III studies to compare goserelin (Zoladex) with orchiectomy and with diethylstilbestrol in treatment of prostatic carcinoma. *Urology* 33 (5 suppl): 45-52.

Perez CA, Hans GE, Leibel SA, Zietman AL, Fuks Z, and Lee WR. 1993. Localized carcinoma of the prostate (stages T1b, T1c, T2, and T3). Review of management with external beam radiation therapy. *Cancer* 72: 3156-73.

Pilepich MV, Sause WT, Shipley WU, Krall JM, et al. 1995. Androgen deprivation with radiation therapy compared with radiation therapy alone for locally advanced prostatic carcinoma: a randomized comparative trial of the radiation therapy oncology group. *Urology* 45: 616-623.

Platt JR, Bree RL, and Schwab RE. 1987. The accuracy of CT in the staging of carcinoma of the prostate. *American Journal of Radiology* 149: 315-8.

Prostate Cancer Trialists' Collaborative Group. 1995. Maximum androgen blockade in advanced prostate cancer: an overview of 22 randomized trials with 3283 deaths in 5710 patients. *Lancet* 346 (8970): 265-269.

Rifkin MD, Zerhouni EA, Gatsonis CA, et al. 1990. Comparison of magnetic resonance imaging and ultrasonography in staging early prostate cancer: Results of a multi-institutional cooperative trial. *New England Journal of Medicine* 323: 621-626.

Rodichok LD, Harper GR, Ruckdeschel JC, Price A, Roberson G, Barron KD, and Horton J. 1981. Early diagnosis of spinal epidural metastases. *American Journal of Medicine* 70: 1181-1188.

Roy CR, Horne D, Raife N, and Pienkos E. 1990. Incidental carcinoma of the prostate: long-term follow-up. *Urology* 36: 210.

Schroder F. 1986. A phase III study of endocrine treatment versus delayed endocrine treatment for patients with pN1-3M0 carcinoma of the prostate. EORTC protocol 30846.

Soloway MS, and Matzkin H. 1993. Antiandrogenic agents as monotherapy in advanced prostatic carcinoma. *Cancer* 71: 1083-8.

Thompson IM, and Zeidman EJ. 1989. Extended follow up of stage A1 carcinoma of the prostate. *Urology* 33: 455.

Top 30 Diagnoses (ICD-9-CM Codes) for Men Ages 65-74 and Men Ages 75+.

Veterans Administrative Cooperative Urological Research Group. 1967. Treatment and survival of patients with cancer of the prostate. *Surgery, Gynecology and Obstetrics* 124: 1011-7.

Vogelzang NJ, Chodak GW, Soloway MS, et al. 1995. Goserelin versus orchiectomy in the treatment of advanced prostate cancer: final results of a randomized trial. *Urology* 46 (2): 220-226.

Whitmore R. 1990. *Urologic Clinics of North America* 17:689.

Zhang G, Wasserman NF, Sidi AM, Reinberg Y, and Reddy PK. 1991. Long-term followup results after expectant management of stage A1 prostatic cancer. *Journal of Urology* 146: 99.

RECOMMENDED QUALITY INDICATORS FOR PROSTATE CANCER TREATMENT

The following criteria apply to men age 18 and older.

	Indicator	Quality of Evidence	Literature	Benefits	Comments
Diagnosis					
1.	A patient *without* any previously known diagnosis of cancer who has an x-ray or radionuclide bone scan with blastic or lytic lesions, or with a notation that the findings are consistent with metastases, should be offered all of the following within the 12 months prior or the 3 weeks following the date of the x-ray or bone scan: a. digital rectal exam; b. PSA.	II-2, III	Leonard and Nystrom, 1993; Hainsworth and Greco, 1993; Huggins, 1941	Reduce prostate cancer morbidity and mortality.	50% of patients with prostate cancer present with bone metastases.
2.	Patients with a new diagnosis of prostate cancer, who have not had a serum PSA in the prior three months, should have serum PSA checked within one month after diagnosis or prior to any treatment, whichever comes first.	II-2, III	Garnick, 1993; Montie, 1996; Partin and Oesterling, 1994; Oesterling, 1993	Reduce prostate cancer morbidity and mortality.	Provides prognostic information and if <10ng/ml, obviates need for bone scan. Only 0.5% of men with PSA less than 10ng/ml had a positive bone scan.
3.	Patients with a new diagnosis of prostate cancer who have a PSA > 10mg/ml should be offered a radionuclide bone scan within 1 month or prior to initiation of any treatment, whichever is first.	II-2, III	Garnick, 1993; Montie, 1996; Partin and Oesterling, 1994; Oesterling, 1993	Reduce morbidity from unnecessary treatment. Target treatment to reduce metastatic prostate cancer morbidity.	Identify patients with metastatic disease. 50% of patients with prostate cancer present with bone metastases.

Indicator	Quality of Evidence	Literature	Benefits	Comments
Treatment				

4. Men *over 60* with minimal prostate cancer (Stage O/A1) should **not** be offered any of the following treatments:
  a. bilateral orchiectomy
  b. LHRH analogue;[1][2]
  c. antiandrogen;[3]
  d. radical prostatectomy;
  e. radiation therapy.
	II-2, III	Epstein, 1986; Lowe, 1988; Roy, 1990; Thompson, 1989; Zhang, 1991	Reduce morbidity from procedure of unproven benefit.	Case series demonstrate survival comparable to general population.

5. Men under 65, who do not have coronary artery disease[4] or a second cancer,[5] should be offered radical prostatectomy or radiation therapy for localized prostate cancer (Stage I & II/A2 & B) within 3 months of staging.	I, II-2, III	Garnick, 1993; Gibbons, 1993; Perez, 1993; Bagshaw et al., 1992, Whitmore, 1990; Adolfsson, 1993; Graversen et al, 1982	Improve survival in selected patients.	Case series suggest similar 10 year survival (85%) for radical prostatectomy, radiation therapy, and observation. While data from randomized controlled trials showing a definite survival benefit for radical prostatectomy or radiation therapy is lacking, most experts would recommend offering such treatment to men with a life expectancy greater than 10 years to provide an option for potential curative therapy.

	Indicator	Quality of Evidence	Literature	Benefits	Comments
6.	Men with metastatic prostate cancer (Stage IV/D) should be offered at least one of the following androgen blockade treatments within three months of staging: • bilateral orchiectomy; • LHRH analogue;[1] • Antiandrogen.[2]	I,III	Garnick, 1993; Daneshgari and Crawford, 1993; Huggins, 1941; VACURG, 1967; Peeling, 1989; Vogelzang , 1995; Kaisary et al. ,1991; EORTC Protocol, 1986; Kirk, 1984; Labrie, 1993; Crawford et al., 1989; Keuppens et al., 1990; Beland et al., 1990;Navaratil, 1987; Janknegt et al., 1993; Bertagna et al., 1994; Prostate Cancer Trialists' Collaborative Group, 1995; Soloway and Matzkin 1993; Pavone-Macaluso et al., 1986; Lund, 1988	Reduce prostate cancer morbidity and mortality.	Randomized controlled trials of bilateral orchiectomy and LHRH analogues have shown them to be equally effective at slowing disease progression. Results are mixed on whether "maximal androgen blockade" with an LHRH analogue and an antiandrogen has a survival benefit over treatment with an LHRH analogue alone. Data regarding monotherapy with antiandrogens is lacking; however, as they have fewer side-effects, they may be appropriate for palliation in some patients.

212

Indicator	Quality of Evidence	Literature	Benefits	Comments
7. Men who undergo orchiectomy for the treatment of prostate cancer should have documented that they were offered treatment with an LHRH analogue or antiandrogen within 12 months prior to surgery.[2]	I, III	Garnick, 1993; Daneshgari and Crawford, 1993; Huggins, 1941; VACURG, 1967; Peeling, 1989; Vogelzang et al., 1995; Kaisary et al., 1991; EORTC, 1986; Kirk, 1984; Labrie et al., 1993;Crawford et al., 1989; Keuppens et al., 1994; Beland et al., 1990; Navaratil, 1987; Janknegt et al., 1994; PCTCG, 1995; Soloway, 1993;Pavone-Macaluso et al., 1986; Lund, 1988	Reduce prostate cancer morbidity.	Randomized controlled trials of bilateral orchiectomy and LHRH analogues have shown them to be equally effective at slowing disease progression.
8. Prostate cancer patients who present with acute low back pain[6] should have documentation within 24 hours of the complaint or in the preceding 3 months of one of the following: • a CT scan of the spine *without* blastic or lytic lesions or compression fractures; • a CT myelogram; • an MRI of the spine.	II-1, III	Osborn et al., 1995; Rodichok et al., 1981; Grant et al., 1994	Reduce prostate cancer morbidity.	Early diagnosis and treatment of cord compression improves functional outcome. 17% false negative rate for cord compression with a normal neurologic exam and normal plain films of the spine.

213

Indicator	Quality of Evidence	Literature	Benefits	Comments
9. Prostate cancer patients with evidence of cord compression on MRI scan of the spine or CT myelogram should be offered one of the following within 24 hours of the radiologic study: • radiation therapy to the spine at a total dose between 3000 cGy and 4500 cGy over 2-4 weeks; • decompressive laminectomy.	I, II-2, III	Osborn et al., 1995; Rodichok et al., 1981; Grant R et al., 1994	Decrease back pain and improve functional outcome.	Case series show benefit for laminectomy followed by radiation therapy over laminectomy alone and no difference between laminectomy and radiation therapy alone.
10. Prostate cancer patients with evidence of cord compression on MRI scan of the spine or CT myelogram should be offered at least 4 mg dexamethazone IV prior to the radiologic study or within 1 hour of its completion, followed by dexamethasone 4 mg IV or PO q six hours for at least 72 hours.	I, II-2, III	Lund & Rasmussen, 1988; Osborn et al., 1995; Rodichok et al., 1981; Grant et al., 1994	Decrease back pain and improve functional outcome.	RCTs of higher doses of dexamethasone have not shown an improvement in neurologic recovery.

214

Definitions and Examples

---

[1] **LHRH Analogue:** The commonly used LHRH analogues in the United States are:
   a. leuprolide (Lupron) 1mg subcutaneous injection daily or 7.5 mg intramuscular injection monthly or 22.3 mg intramuscular injection every 3 months
   b. goserelin acetate (Zoladex) 3.6 mg depot injection monthly or 10.8 mg depot injection every 3 months

[2] **Antiandrogen:** The antiandrogens commonly used in the United States include
   a. flutamide (Eulexin) 250 mg by mouth three times a day
   b. bicalutamide (Casodex) 50 mg by mouth daily
   c. nilutamide (Anandron) 300 mg by mouth daily for the first month of treatment followed by 150 mg by mouth daily thereafter

[3] **Coronary Artery Disease:** A person shall be considered to have coronary artery disease if he has any of the following documented in the chart in progress notes, problem lists, or as discharge diagnoses:
   a. coronary artery disease
   b. angina
   c. myocardial infarction
   d. coronary artery bypass graft surgery
   e. PTCA
   f. congestive heart failure
   g. a coronary angiogram with at least one vessel with an occlusion >70%

[4] **Second Cancer:** A person shall be considered to have a second cancer if he has any of the following documented in the chart in progress notes, problem lists, or as discharge diagnoses:
   a. any cancer other than prostate cancer except for basal cell and squamous cell skin cancers
   b. treatment with chemotherapy

[6] **Acute low back pain:** No record of chronic low back pain pre-dating the prostate cancer diagnosis.

Quality of Evidence Codes

I	RCT
II-1	Nonrandomized controlled trials
II-2	Cohort or case analysis
II-3	Multiple time series
III	Opinions or descriptive studies

215

10. SKIN CANCER SCREENING

Patricia Bellas, MD

In this chapter we will address cutaneous melanoma (CM) and nonmelanoma skin cancers (NMSC) including basal cell (BCC) and squamous cell (SCC) cancers. We will not address vulvar or penile cancer specifically nor will we address other rarer skin cancers. The USPSTF report *Guide to Preventive Services, 2nd edition* (USPSTF, 1996) and several other recent review articles (Preston and Stern, 1992; Marks, 1996; Marks, 1995; NIH, 1992; Koh, Geller, Miller, Grossbart, and Lew, 1996; Rhodes, 1995) obtained from a MEDLINE search formed the basis of this chapter. In addition, we performed a supplementary brief review of recently published books dealing with melanoma prevention and a 1993 to 1996 MEDLINE search of articles on skin cancer prevention (Meyer, et al., 1996; MacKie, 1996; Berwick, Begg, Fine, Roush, and Barnhill, 1996; Black, et al., 1995).

IMPORTANCE

There are an estimated 800,000 new cases of skin cancer diagnosed each year in the US. More than 95 percent of these cancers are NMSC, accounting for approximately one-third of all cancers diagnosed in the US. Although metastasis is uncommon in NMSC, resulting in 2100 deaths per year, there remains significant morbidity from local tissue destruction, and medical costs probably exceed $500 million annually. The mean age of onset is 60 to 65 (USPSTF, 1996; Preston and Stern, 1992).

Cutaneous melanoma (CM) comprises an estimated 34,100 annual incident cases annually, and 7200 deaths. Nearly half of all these cancer deaths occurred in men over 50. The incidence of CM in whites is higher (9.2 per 100,000) than in Hispanics (1.9 per 100,000) or in African Americans and Asians (0.7 to 1.2 per 100,000). There is concern however that the incidence is increasing. It ranks second among adult onset cancers in years of potential life lost as its median age of diagnosis is 53. It is the seventh most frequent cancer in whites in the US (more common than ovarian, cervical, CNS, and leukemia) (USPSTF, 1996; Marks, 1995).

Epidemiologic data and experimental evidence support cumulative sun exposure (especially UV B radiation) as the major risk for NMSC (Preston and Stern, 1992). Additional factors include: age; a previous NMSC (about 50 percent of patients with a history of NMSC will develop a new skin cancer within five years); a sun sensitive skin type with freckling, relative inability to tan (Indicator 1); light skin and hair color; immunocompromised state (e.g., renal transplant patients in one study had a 253-fold risk of SCC and a tenfold risk of BCC); chemical carcinogens (arsenic, psoralens and UVA treatment, coal tar products and cigarette smoke); ionizing radiation; chronic ulceration or inflammation; viral (HPV); and certain genodermatoses[1] (USPSTF, 1996; Preston and Stern, 1992). SCC precursors include solar keratoses (AKs) which are fairly prevalent in the population; about one in 1000 per year progress to invasive cancer (Sober and Burstein, 1995). There has also been a hypothesized link to high fat diet in association with UV radiation exposure (Black, et al., 1995).

CM risk factors, besides white race, with a relative risk of eight or more include: Familial Atypical Mole and Melanoma syndrome; melanocytic precursors or marker lesions including multiple typical moles,[2] atypical moles[3] and specific congenital moles; prior CM, or CM in a first degree relative (Rhodes, 1995). Additional lower order risk factors include a history of severe sunburn; ease of burning/inability to tan; light hair or blue eyes; family history of NMSC; and excessive sun exposure. The relationship with solar radiation is less clear than with NMSC, although there is some evidence that infrequent, intense exposure (blistering sunburn) at a young age may be linked to CM (Rhodes, 1995) (Indicators 1 and 3).

---

[1] Genodermatoses: Certain genetic skin conditions. Those syndromes most commonly associated with a high risk of NMSC include Xeroderma Pigmentosum, Basal-cell nevus syndrome, Albinism, and Epidermodysplasia

[2] Quantitative examples of multiple common moles include counts of 50 nevi >= 2 mm diameter, or 5 nevi >=5 mm diameter.

[3] Also referred to as dysplastic nevi.

SCREENING

Primary prevention interventions include two strategies:

(1) Public education programs

These focus on midday sun avoidance and use of protective clothing (hats, etc.) and use of sunscreens. There is fair evidence that sun avoidance during the midday is effective in preventing skin cancer, while use of sunscreens is controversial. A RCT showed some sunscreens (UVA and UVB blocking agents) effective in preventing new AKs (Thompson, Jolley, and Marks, 1993) but there is conflicting data regarding prevention of NMSC or CM. The USPSTF gives avoidance of sun exposure and the use of protective clothing for adults at risk of skin cancer a "B" recommendation with a "C" recommendation for sunscreen use – insufficient evidence to counsel for or against, except perhaps for persons with solar keratoses (USPSTF, 1996) (Indicator 2).

(2) Clinician counseling

This targets high risk persons to reduce sun exposure through the previously mentioned means. There is some limited evidence that physician counseling regarding sun avoidance can lead to behavior change (USPSTF, 1996). The ACS, AAD, AMA and NIH Consensus Panel recommend patient education on sun avoidance and use of sunscreens (SPF 15 or higher). The USPSTF recommends counseling patients at risk of skin cancer on sun avoidance as does the AAFP (Indicators 1, 2 and 3). One recently published RCT documented the efficacy of a low fat diet in decreasing new NMSC over a two year period in patients with a previous NMSC; however, no indicators are recommended at this time (Black, et al., 1995).

Secondary prevention or early detection of lesions has been approached by three strategies:

(1) Self-examination

This involves promoting regular skin self-examination and disseminating information regarding what constitutes a suspicious lesion or lesion change through public programs or clinician counseling. Skin self-examination can be used for early detection of skin cancer and for evaluating risk status (number of moles, unusual moles). The American Cancer Society has promulgated the "ABCDs" of pigmented lesions as warning signs to seek medical care ("A" is for asymmetry, "B" is border irregularity, "C" is color variegation and "D" is for large diameter [over 6 mm]). A recent population-based case control study (Thompson, Jolley, and Marks, 1993) found that skin self-examination was associated with a reduced risk of melanoma incidence (OR 0.66, 95% CI 0.44-0.99) and that it may reduce the risk of advanced disease among melanoma patients. The authors recommended a longer follow-up study to verify this claim. The American Cancer Society recommends monthly skin self-examination for all adults, with physician skin exams every three years for persons age 20 to 39 and yearly in persons over age 40. The USPSTF gives a "C" recommendation (insufficient evidence) to counseling patients to perform periodic skin self-examination, except for those with established risk factors for skin cancer (Indicators 4 and 5).

(2) Clinician screening

The goal of physical examination of the skin by a clinician is detection of any suspicious lesion, which should then be confirmed by biopsy. No indicators relating to biopsy are recommended, however, since documentation of lesion characteristics is likely to be inadequate. Among patients presenting for a free skin screening by dermatologists, the sensitivity of the visual exam was 89 to 97 percent with a predictive positive value of 35 to 75 percent for skin cancer (Koh, Geller, Miller, Grossbart, and Lew, 1996). A more recent evaluation of the American Academy of Dermatology (AAD) skin cancer screening programs found the positive predictive value was only seven percent (Koh, et al., 1996). Compared to dermatologists, non-dermatologists are less likely to be able to correctly identify skin lesions from color photographs (USPSTF, 1996). Furthermore, interobserver reliability in identifying atypical moles is poor, although evaluating the numbers and size of moles is more reliable (Meyer, et al., 1996). Although NMSC are common, there is no strong evidence that lesions found by screening result in better outcomes. Theoretically, lesions discovered early should be easier to treat with less disfigurement (USPSTF, 1996). Screening for CM by primary care providers has also not been shown to lead to reduced morbidity and mortality in this country. A time series study in Scotland showed an upward trend in thin tumor presentation and a trend toward decrease in the mortality rate (for women, but not for men) 15 years after a public and professional education program targeting primary care physicians (MacKie, 1996).

There are no published data evaluating the optimum frequency of screening or surveillance. The USPSTF gives routine screening by primary care providers using a total skin exam a "C" recommendation, indicating there is insufficient evidence to recommend for or against it. Opportunistic screening or case finding, which involves sporadic clinician skin examination of patients who present for another medical problem, is encouraged. However, we are not recommending quality indicators for this.

(3) Surveillance

Surveillance involves regular examination of individuals with previously demonstrated high risk of melanoma or NMSC. Several studies (time series and cohort) have shown that high risk populations under surveillance of dermatologists, often using photography, have tumors discovered at a thinner level than tumors found in the general population or in the index cases (MacKie et al., 1993; Koh, Geller et al., 1996). For CM, there is fairly good evidence that detection and excision at an early stage has a better prognosis. If at time of excision the tumor thickness is less than 0.76 mm, the ten year survival rate is more than 95 percent. If the tumor thickness is greater than 4 mm there is less than a 50 percent ten year survival rate (Rhodes, 1995). The USPSTF recommends that providers consider referring specific high risk persons to skin cancer specialists for surveillance (Indicator 6). In addition, the NIH consensus panel also recommends that all melanoma patients be enrolled in surveillance and a careful family history be taken. High risk family members should also be enrolled in surveillance (Indicators 7, 8, and 9).

In summary, expert opinion and observational data support efforts to reduce skin cancer incidence, morbidity, and mortality by putting emphasis on both public education and an individual approach directed at high risk persons such as the elderly. Clinician strategies include recommending sun protection, promoting skin cancer awareness, and using opportunistic case finding to detect skin cancer and identify very high risk persons for surveillance.

REFERENCES

Berwick M, Begg C, Fine J, Roush G, and Barnhill R. 3 January 1996. Screening for cutaneous melanoma by skin self-examination. *Journal of the National Cancer Institute* 88 (1): 17-23.

Black H, et al. 1995. Evidence that a low-fat diet reduces the occurrence of non-melanoma skin cancer. *International Journal of Cancer* 62: 165-169.

Koh H, et al. 1996. Evaluation of the American Academy of Dermatology's national skin cancer early detection and screening program. *Journal of the American Academy of Dermatology* 34: 971-8.

Koh H, Geller A, Miller D, Grossbart T, and Lew R. April 1996. Prevention and early detection strategies for melanoma and skin cancer. *Archives of Dermatology* 132: 436-443.

MacKie R. 11 May 1996. *Pigment Cell. Primary and secondary prevention of malignant melanoma.* Switzerland: KargerBasek.

MacKie R, McHenry P, and Hole D. 26 June 1993. Accelerated detection with prospective surveillance for cutaneous malignant melanoma in high-risk groups. *Lancet* 341 (1618-20):

Marks R. 15 January 1995. An Overview of skin Cancers. Incidence and Causation. *Cancer* 75 (2 Suppl): 607-12.

Marks R. 1996. Prevention and Control of Melanoma: The public health approach. *CA Cancer Journal for Clinicians* 46 (4): 199-216.

Meyer LJ, et al. 1996. Interobserver concordance in discriminating clinical atypia of melanocytic nevi, and correlations with histologic atypia. *Journal of the American Academy of Dermatology* 34: 618-25.

NIH Consensus Conference. 9 September 1992. Diagnosis and treatment of early melanoma. *Journal of the American Medical Association* 268 (10): 1314-9.

Preston DS, and Stern RS. 3 December 1992. Nonmelanoma cancers of the skin. *New England Journal of Medicine* 327 (23): 1649-62.

Rhodes AR. 15 January 1995. Public education and cancer of the skin. What do people need to know about melanoma and nonmelanoma skin cancer? *Cancer* 75 (2 Suppl): 613-36.

Sober AJ, and Burstein JM. 15 January 1995. Precursors to skin cancer. *Cancer* 75 (2 Suppl): 645-50.

Thompson SC, Jolley D, and Marks R. 1993. Reduction of solar keratoses by regular sunscreen use. *New England Journal of Medicine* 329: 1147-1151.

US Preventative Services Task Force. 1996. *Guide to Clinical Preventative Services, 2nd ed.* Baltimore: Williams & Wilkins.

RECOMMENDED QUALITY INDICATORS FOR SKIN CANCER SCREENING

The following indicators apply to men and women age 18 and older.

Indicator	Quality of Evidence	Literature	Benefits	Comments
Primary Prevention				
1. When a patient is noted to have a sunburn, the chart should document counseling regarding avoidance of midday sun, use of protective clothing, and/or use of sunscreens.	III II-2 II-3[1]	NIH Consensus Panel, 1992	Prevent skin cancer.	People who have a sunburn are not practicing skin protection and most likely are in a higher risk group for skin cancer.
2. Patients who have evidence of aktinic keratosis or solar keratosis (AK)[2], should be counseled regarding avoidance of midday sun, use of protective clothing, and/or use of sunscreens within 1 year before or after diagnosis.	I, III II-2 II-3[1]	Thompson, USPSTF; 1996	Prevent development of new AKs. Prevent skin cancer.	AKs are considered precursors for squamous cell carcinoma.
3. All patients noted to have strong skin cancer risk factors[3] should be instructed in midday sun avoidance, use of protective clothing, and/or use of sunscreens within 1 year before or after note of high risk.	III II-2 II-3[1]	USPSTF 1996	Prevent skin cancer.	
Secondary Prevention/Skin Self-exam				
4. All patients noted to have strong skin cancer risk factors[3] should be instructed in skin self-examination within 1 year before or after note of high risk.	II-2, III	Berwick, 1996; USPSTF, 1996	Prevent morbidity and mortality by looking for melanoma or melanocytic precursor or marker lesions.	Lesions detected early may have a better prognosis.

Indicator	Quality of Evidence	Literature	Benefits	Comments
5. All patients with a personal history of melanoma or non-melanoma skin cancer (NMSC) should be counseled to do skin self-examination within 1 year before or after the history is documented.	II, III	NIH Consensus Panel, 1992; Berwick, 1996	Prevent morbidity and mortality by looking for melanoma or melanocytic precursor or marker lesions.	Lesions detected early may have a better prognosis.
Secondary Prevention/Clinician Screening				
6. Patients diagnosed with NMSC or multiple AKs[2] in the past 5 years should have a skin exam documented in the past 12 months.	III	Preston, 1992; ACS, AAD, AAFP, 1996	Prevent morbidity and mortality from skin cancer.	Lesions detected early may have a better prognosis. About 50% of patients will develop a new skin cancer within 5 years.
7. Referral to a dermatologist for surveillance/screening should be documented if a patient has either of the following: a. personal history of cutaneous melanoma (CM),[4] b. multiple common or atypical moles[5] plus a family history of CM (possible FAM-M phenotype[6]).	II-2, II-3 III	MacKie, 1994; NIH Consensus Panel, 1992; USPSTF, 1996	Prevent morbidity and mortality by looking for melanoma or melanocytic precursor or marker lesions.	Melanoma lesions, when detected in patients under surveillance, tend to be thinner. Thinner lesions have a better prognosis.
8. All patients newly diagnosed with melanoma should be advised to have family members undergo a screening skin exam.	III	NIH Consensus Panel, 1996	Prevent morbidity and mortality by looking for melanoma or melanocytic precursor or marker lesions.	Although uncommon, the genetic phenotype associated with melanoma conveys a very high risk.
9. All patients with a documented family history of melanoma in a first degree relative should have a screening skin exam at least once in the year preceding or subsequent to documentation.	III	NIH Consensus Panel, 1996	Prevent morbidity and mortality by looking for melanoma or melanocytic precursor or marker lesions.	See above.

225

Definitions and Examples

[1] II-2 and II-3 for indicators 1-3 relate to evidence linking sun exposure to these cancers, though there is no evidence directly linking protective measures and decreased rates of skin cancer.

[2] AKs: aktinic keratosis or solar keratosis. These are both a precursor and a marker of increased risk for NMSC. Clinically, they are rough, scaly, erythematious patches on chronically sun exposed skin.

[3] Strong skin cancer risk factors: family history of skin cancer, large number of moles, or atypical moles. [5]

[4] Cutaneous melanoma.

[5] Atypical moles: Also referred to in the literature as dysplastic nevi, these are acquired pigmented lesions of the skin; they vary in size, have macular and/or papular components and have borders that usually are irregular and frequently ill defined. Their color is variegated. Histologically they exhibit architectural disorder, with or without melanocytic atypia. Atypical nevi may occur in 5-10% of the population.

[6] FAM-M: Familial atypical mole and melanoma syndrome - a syndrome characterized by the occurance of melanoma in one or more first degree or second degree relatives, plus having a large number of moles (often > 50) and moles with distinct histologic features; lifetime risk of development of melanoma may approach 100%.

Quality of Evidence Codes

I	Randomized Controlled Trial (RCT)
II-1	Nonrandomized controlled trials
II-2	Cohort or case analysis
II-3	Multiple time series
III	Opinions or descriptive studies

226

11. CANCER PAIN AND PALLIATION

Jennifer Reifel, M.D.

While supportive care was not one of the original clinical areas selected for the development of quality indicators, the Oncology and HIV Panel felt that this was a significant omission. Based upon the panel's recommendations, the staff drafted four indicators for cancer pain management and the treatment of vomiting. The panel accepted two indicators for pain management and one indicator for the prevention of chemotherapy-induced emesis. The core references for this chapter include a chapter on cancer pain in the textbook *Supportive Care* (Cherny, 1998), the AHCPR (Jacox et al., 1994) and ASCO (1992) clinical practice guidelines for the management of cancer pain, and the National Cancer Institute (1997) statement on the management nausea and vomiting from CancerNet PDQ Information for Health Care Professionals.

CANCER PAIN

Importance

Cancer is diagnosed in over 1 million Americans each year. Approximately 8 million Americans either currently have cancer or have a history of cancer (Jacox et al., 1994). The prevalence of pain in patients newly diagnosed with cancer is approximately 30 percent. In patients with advanced disease, the prevalence of pain approaches 80 percent (Cherny, 1998). Among cancer patients with pain, 40 to 50 percent report it to be moderate to severe and an additional 25 to 30 percent describe it as very severe (Jacox et al., 1994).

Diagnosis

Cancer pain is frequently undertreated and the most important reason for this is inadequate assessment (Jacox et al., 1994; Cherny, 1998.). Studies have shown that the most important predictor of inadequate pain relief is a discrepancy between the patient's and physician's evaluation of the severity of the pain (Cherny, 1998; Jacox et al., 1994). For this reason, the AHCPR Guideline makes this recommendation: "Health professionals should ask about pain, and the patient's self-report should be the primary source of assessment" (Jacox et al., 1994).

Initial pain assessment should include a description of its character and intensity (Cherny, 1998; Jacox et al., 1994; ASCO 1992). Pain rating scales can be useful adjuncts to patient's qualitative description of the pain and are recommended in the AHCPR and ASCO guidelines (Jacox et al., 1994; ASCO, 1992). In addition, a complete physical exam, as well as appropriate diagnostic tests, should be performed to attempt to localize the pain and determine its cause (Cherny, 1998; Jacox et al., 1994; ASCO, 1992).

Pain associated with cancer can have many etiologies. Acute pain may be the result of diagnostic or therapeutic procedures, anticancer therapies (such as the intravenous infusion of chemotherapy), infections, or paraneoplastic complications (such as thromboses). Most chronic cancer pain is caused by the local effects of the tumor on bones or nerves. Bone metastases are the most common cause of chronic pain in cancer patients (Cherny, 1998).

Based upon the these guidelines and the advice of our expert panel, we proposed, and the panel accepted, a quality indicator that requires an assessment of cancer pain at least once every six months for all patients with cancer metastatic to bone (Jacox et al., 1994; ASCO 1992) (Indicator 1). While all cancer patients should be vigilantly evaluated for pain on an ongoing basis, this indicator is limited to patients with metastases to bone since this well-defined group has the highest prevalence of cancer pain. Furthermore, in the absence of published guidelines on the frequency of pain assessment, we have selected every six months as a *minimum* requirement.

Treatment

Cancer pain can be controlled in approximately 90 percent of patients with standard analgesic therapy (Jacox et al., 1994). The World Health Organization has developed a well-validated and widely accepted analgesic ladder for the effective titration of pain medications in cancer patients (WHO, 1996; Berger et al., 1998; Jacox et al., 1994; ASCO 1992). This analgesic ladder has three steps. The first step, for mild pain, is a non-steroidal analgesic medication (NSAID). For moderate pain, or pain that does not respond to step one, the clinician should move to step two: a weak opioid, such as codeine or hydrocodone, in combination with an NSAID. Patients with severe pain, or pain that is not relieved by the step two approach, should be treated with step three medications: strong opioid drugs such as morphine, hydromorphone, methadone, or fentanyl. The opioid doses should be increased as needed to control pain. Based on the WHO approach, and AHCPR and ASCO guidelines, we proposed an indicator requiring that cancer patients whose pain is uncontrolled be offered a change in pain management within 24 hours of the pain complaint (Jacox et al., 1994; ASCO 1992) (Indicator 2). The panel accepted this indicator.

Palliative radiation therapy is an important adjuvant to the pharmacological treatment of pain. Radiation therapy is indicated in the treatment of symptomatic metastases where tumor infiltration has caused pain, compression, bleeding or obstruction (Jacox et al., 1994; Cherny, 1998). The treatment of bony metastases with localized radiation therapy results in at least partial relief of symptoms in over 70 percent of patients (Jacox et al., 1994; Berger et al., 1998). However, the effectiveness and durability of radiation therapy in producing pain relief is dependent upon the location of the tumor as well as the type (some tumors are less radiosensitive.) In addition to external beam radiation, systemic radioisotopes, such as Strontium-89, are also available. Systemic radioisotopes provide an attractive alternative for patients with widely disseminated bone metastases (Jacox et al., 1994; Berger et al., 1998). The AHCPR Guideline recommends that non-invasive pharmacologic analgesic therapies be attempted prior to the more invasive approach required with radiation therapy. The Oncology and HIV Expert Panel considered a quality indicator specifying that patients with painful bony metastases, who are unresponsive to or intolerant of narcotic analgesia, should be offered radiation therapy or Strontium-89 within one week (Indicator 3). This indicator was dropped by the panel due to low validity and feasibility scores.

CHEMOTHERAPY ASSOCIATED EMESIS

Importance

Prevention and treatment of nausea and vomiting in cancer patients is of paramount importance as the symptom can lead to serious metabolic derangements, deterioration of physical and mental well-being, decreased functional status, and withdrawal from potentially curative treatment. (National Cancer Institute, 1997) Five different emesis syndromes have been identified and described in patients receiving chemotherapy:

1. *Acute chemotherapy-induced emesis* is defined as nausea and vomiting that occurs within the 24-hour period immediately following chemotherapy administration.

2. *Delayed emesis* begins after the first 24-hours following chemotherapy.

3. *Anticipatory emesis* is a behaviorally conditioned response that occurs prior to subsequent chemotherapy in response to a stimulus (such as the nurse starting the intravenous line.)

4. *Breakthrough emesis* is vomiting that occurs on the day of chemotherapy in spite of appropriate prophylaxis.

5. *Refractory emesis* is vomiting that occurs despite optimal antiemetic treatment in previous course (Cherny, 1998).

The most important factor in determining whether a patient experiences nausea and vomiting with chemotherapy is the emetogenicity of the chemotherapy (Hasketh et al., 1997; National Cancer Institute, 1997; Cherny, 1998). Chemotherapy agents are classified according to their emetogenic potential, based upon the percentage of patients who will experience emesis with that drug administered as a single agent (Hasketh et al., 1997; National Cancer Institute, 1997; Cherny, 1998). In addition, the potential for emesis with most chemotherapy agents increases with increasing dose and can often be worsened when it is given in combination with other agents (Hasketh et al., 1997).

Treatment

There are many drugs available to treat chemotherapy associated emesis, including prochlorperazine, metoclopromide, lorazepam, and steroids. However, the use of highly selective antagonists of the type 3 serotonin receptor has had the greatest impact on controlling symptoms from highly emetogenic chemotherapy. In randomized controlled trials, the serotonin antagonists have demonstrated equal or superior efficacy to high dose metoclopromide, with fewer side effects, for acute chemotherapy-induced emesis (National Cancer Institute, 1997; Cherny, 1998). However, studies of serotonin antagonists for the treatment of delayed chemotherapy-induced emesis have not shown them to have an advantage over conventional therapies (National Cancer Institute, 1997; Cherny, 1998). The FDA indication for intravenous preparations of serotonin antagonist anti-emetics is limited to the prophylaxis of chemotherapy-induced emesis in the setting of highly emetogenic chemotherapy (National Cancer Institute, 1997).

Consistent with the literature, we proposed a quality indicator requiring that all patients receiving highly or severely emetogenic chemotherapy (see Table 11.1) be offered concurrent type 3 selective serotonin antagonist anti-emetic therapy (Indicator 4).

Table 11.1
Severely and Highly Emetogenic Chemotherapy Agents

Severely Emetogenic Agents	Highly Emetogenic Agents
Carmustine (>250 mg/m^2)	Carboplatin
Cisplatin (>50 mg/m^2)	Carmustine (<250 mg/m^2)
Cyclophosphamide (>1500 mg/m^2)	Cisplatin (<50 mg/m^2)
Dacarbazine	Cyclophosphamide
Mechlorethamine	(>700 mg/m^2 and <1500 mg/m^2)
Streptozocin	Cytarabine (>1g/m^2)
	Doxorubicin (>60 mg/m^2)
	Methotrexate (>1000 mg/m^2)
	Procarbazine

Source: Adapted from Heskath et al., 1997

REFERENCES

Ad Hoc Committee on Cancer Pain of the Society of Clinical Oncology. 1992. Cancer Pain Assessment and Treatment Curriculum Guidelines. *Journal of Clinical Oncology* 10:1976-1982.

Cherny NI. Cancer Pain: Principles of Assessment and Syndromes in *Supportive Care,* Berger A, Portenoy RK, and Weissman DE, eds. Lippincott-Raven, 1998. Philadelphia, PA.

Heskath PJ, Kris MG, Grunber SM, Beck T, et al. 1997. Proposal for classifying the acute emetogenicity of cancer chemotherapy. *Journal of Clinical Oncology* 15:103-109.

Jacox A, Carr DB, Payne R, et al. March 1994. *Management of Cancer Pain. Clinical Practice Guideline No. 9.* AHCPR Publication No. 94-0592. Agency for Health Care Policy and Research, U.S. Department of Health and Human Services, Public Health Service, Rockville, Maryland.

Janjan NA and Weissman DE. Primary Cancer Treatment: Antineoplastic Syndromes in *Supportive Care,* Berger A, Portenoy RK, and Weissman DE, eds. Lippincott-Raven, 1998. Philadelphia, PA.

National Cancer Institute. June 1997. Nausea and Vomiting. CancerNet PDQ Information on Supportive Care for Health Care Professionals.

Payne R. Pharmacologic Management of Pain Syndromes in *Supportive Care,* Berger A, Portenoy RK, and Weissman DE, eds. Lippincott-Raven, 1998. Philadelphia, PA.

Pisters KMW and Kris MG. Treatment-related Nausea and Vomiting Syndromes in *Supportive Care,* Berger A, Portenoy RK, and Weissman DE, eds. Lippincott-Raven, 1998. Philadelphia, PA.

World Health Organization (WHO). Cancer pain relief: With a guide to opioid availability, Second Edition. 1996.

RECOMMEDED QUALITY INDICATORS FOR CANCER PAIN AND PALLIATION

The following indicators apply to men and women age 18 and older.

Indicator	Quality of Evidence	Literature	Benefits	Comments
Diagnosis				
1. Patients with metastatic cancer to bone should have the presence or absence of pain noted at least every 6 months.	II-2, II	Jacox et al., 1994; ASCO, 1992	Improve pain management.	While all cancer patients should have their pain addressed, we have limited this quality indicator to patients with bony metastases since this is the group with the highest prevalence of pain.
Treatment				
2. Cancer patients whose pain is uncontrolled should be offered a change in pain management within 24 hours of the pain complaint.	III	Jacox et al., 1994; ASCO, 1992	Reduce pain.	Cancer pain can be controlled in 90% of patients with standard analgesic therapy.
3. Patients with painful bony metastases, who are noted to be unresponsive to or intolerant of narcotic analgesia, should be offered one of the following within one week of the notation of pain: • Radiation therapy to the sites of pain; • radioactive strontium therapy.	II-1, II-2, III	Jacox et al., 1994	Reduce pain.	70% of patients with painful bony metastases will have at least partial relief of symptoms with radiation therapy.
4. Patients receiving emetogenic chemotherapy should be offered concurrent potent antiemetic therapy (e.g. 5HT blockade).[1]	I, III, III	National Cancer Institute, 1997	Reduce emesis.	In RCTs, serotonin antagonists have demonstrated superior efficacy to metoclopromide.

Definitions and Examples

[1] Potent antiemetic therapy: Ondansetron (Zofran), granisetron (Kytrel), dolasetron mesylate, tropisetron, batanopride.

Quality of Evidence Codes

I	Randomized Controlled Trial (RCT)
II-1	Nonrandomized controlled trials
II-2	Cohort or case analysis
II-3	Multiple time series
III	Opinions or descriptive studies

APPENDIX A: PANEL RATING SHEETS BY CONDITION

APPENDIX A: PANEL RATING SHEETS BY CONDITION

	Validity	Feasibility

1. Women aged 50-70 should have had a screening mammography performed at least every 2 years.

INDICATOR ADDED AFTER ROUND 1

```
               1   1 7            1   8
1 2 3 4 5 6 7 8 9  1 2 3 4 5 6 7 8 9  ( 1- 2)
  (9.0, 0.4, A)      (9.0, 0.2, A)
```

2. Women aged 50-70 should have a clinical breast exam of both breasts at least every 2 years.

```
   1 2 2 4            1   2 3 3
1 2 3 4 5 6 7 8 9  1 2 3 4 5 6 7 8 9  ( 3- 4)
  (6.0, 0.9, I)      (8.0, 0.9, A)
```

Scales: 1 = low validity or feasibility; 9 = high validity or feasibility

NOTE: This chapter includes indicators previously rated for Q1. Only new or revised indicators are being rated.

TREATMENT

5. Women with stage I or stage II breast cancer should be offered a choice of modified radical mastectomy or breast-conserving surgery, unless contraindications to breast-conserving surgery are present.

```
                    1 2 6            1 1 2 1 1 3
          1 2 3 4 5 6 7 8 9  1 2 3 4 5 6 7 8 9   ( 1- 2)
            (9.0, 0.4, A)       (7.0, 1.6, I)
```

6. Women treated with breast conserving surgery should begin radiation therapy within 6 weeks of completing either of the following (unless wound complications prevent the initiation of treatment):

- last surgical procedure on the breast (including reconstructive surgery that occurs within 6 weeks of primary resection)
- chemotherapy, if patient receives adjuvant chemotherapy

```
                      4   5             3 6
          1 2 3 4 5 6 7 8 9  1 2 3 4 5 6 7 8 9   ( 3- 4)
            (9.0, 0.9, A)       (9.0, 0.3, A)
```

7. Women with invasive breast cancer that is node positive, or node-negative and primary tumor >=1cm, should be treated with adjuvant systemic therapy to include at least one of the following:

- Combination chemotherapy (more than one agent, lasting for at least 2 months).
- Tamoxifen (20mg/d for at least 2 years).

```
                    4 2 3             1 4 4
          1 2 3 4 5 6 7 8 9  1 2 3 4 5 6 7 8 9   ( 5- 6)
            (8.0, 0.8, A)       (8.0, 0.6, A)
```

FOLLOW-UP

8. Women with a history of breast cancer should have yearly mammography.

```
                      1   8                 9
          1 2 3 4 5 6 7 8 9  1 2 3 4 5 6 7 8 9   ( 7- 8)
            (9.0, 0.2, A)       (9.0, 0.0, A)
```

9. Women diagnosed with breast cancer in the past 5 years should have a clinical breast exam at least once a year.

```
          1         2 1 5               3 6
          1 2 3 4 5 6 7 8 9  1 2 3 4 5 6 7 8 9   ( 9- 10)
            (9.0, 1.3, A)       (9.0, 0.3, A)
```

10. Women diagnosed with breast cancer more than 5 years ago should have a clinical breast exam at least once a year.

```
          1         1 3 4               4 5
          1 2 3 4 5 6 7 8 9  1 2 3 4 5 6 7 8 9   ( 11- 12)
            (8.0, 1.2, A)       (9.0, 0.4, A)
```

INDICATOR ADDED AFTER ROUND 1

11. Women with metastatic breast cancer should be offered at least one of the following treatments within 6 weeks of the identification of metastases:

- Hormonal therapy
- Chemotherapy
- Enrollment in a clinical trial with documentation of informed consent

```
                    1 4 4             1 3 5
          1 2 3 4 5 6 7 8 9  1 2 3 4 5 6 7 8 9   ( 13- 14)
            (8.0, 0.6, A)       (9.0, 0.6, A)
```

Scales: 1 = low validity or feasibility; 9 = high validity or feasibility

INDICATOR ADDED AFTER ROUND 1

4. Women with a history of cervical
dysplasia, carcinoma-in-situ or HIV infection
should have a pap smear performed at least   1 4 4   1 1 7
once a year.   1 2 3 4 5 6 7 8 9 1 2 3 4 5 6 7 8 9 (1- 2)
                                            (8.0, 0.6, A)   (9.0, 0.3, A)

1. Patients documented in the chart as
having one or more first degree relatives
with CRC should be offered at least one of
the following colon cancer screening test
beginning at age 40:
  - FOBT (if not done in the past 2 years)
  - Sigmoidoscopy (if not done in the past
    5 years)
  - Colonoscopy (if not done in the past 10
    years)
  - Double contrast barium enema
    (if not done in the past 5 years)

```
                         1 4 4                  2 3 4
             1 2 3 4 5 6 7 8 9    1 2 3 4 5 6 7 8 9   ( 1- 2)
               (8.0, 0.6, A)        (8.0, 0.7, A)
```

3. Providers should offer to remove all
polyps with either of the following
characteristics within 3 months of detection:

  a. size greater than 1 cm

```
                         4 2 3                  2 4 3
             1 2 3 4 5 6 7 8 9    1 2 3 4 5 6 7 8 9   ( 3- 4)
               (8.0, 0.8, A)        (8.0, 0.6, A)
```

  b. adenomatous histology

```
                         4 2 3                  2 4 3
             1 2 3 4 5 6 7 8 9    1 2 3 4 5 6 7 8 9   ( 5- 6)
               (8.0, 0.8, A)        (8.0, 0.6, A)
```

5. Surveillance colonoscopy should not be
repeated sooner than 3 years following the
removal of adenomatous polyps in otherwise
average risk patients.

```
                       1 4 2 2                4 1 4
             1 2 3 4 5 6 7 8 9    1 2 3 4 5 6 7 8 9   ( 7- 8)
               (7.0, 0.8, A)        (8.0, 0.9, A)
```

6. Procedure note documentation for
endoscopic management of polyps should
include:

  a. Whether biopsy only versus complete
     removal of polyps was performed

```
                         3 4 2                1 1     7
             1 2 3 4 5 6 7 8 9    1 2 3 4 5 6 7 8 9   ( 9- 10)
               (8.0, 0.6, A)        (9.0, 0.6, A)
```

  b. Location of any polyps removed
     endoscopically

```
                         2 3 4                2     7
             1 2 3 4 5 6 7 8 9    1 2 3 4 5 6 7 8 9   ( 11- 12)
               (8.0, 0.7, A)        (9.0, 0.4, A)
```

  c. Polyp type: sessile versus pedunculated

```
                         3 4 2                2 1 6
             1 2 3 4 5 6 7 8 9    1 2 3 4 5 6 7 8 9   ( 13- 14)
               (8.0, 0.6, A)        (9.0, 0.6, A)
```

7. All patients with positive screening
sigmoidoscopy tests should be offered a
diagnostic colonoscopy within 3 months.

```
                         1 5 3                  2 3 4
             1 2 3 4 5 6 7 8 9    1 2 3 4 5 6 7 8 9   ( 15- 16)
               (8.0, 0.4, A)        (8.0, 0.7, A)
```

8. If a screening FOBT is positive, a
diagnostic evaluation of the colon should be
offered within a 3 month period.

```
             1             5 3                  2 3 4
             1 2 3 4 5 6 7 8 9    1 2 3 4 5 6 7 8 9   ( 17- 18)
               (8.0, 1.0, A)        (8.0, 0.7, A)
```

9. A FOBT should be offered to those who
refuse other screening tests for CRC.

```
             5           2 1 1 3        1     1 2 2
             1 2 3 4 5 6 7 8 9    1 2 3 4 5 6 7 8 9   ( 19- 20)
               (1.0, 3.0, D)        (7.0, 2.9, D)
```

10. All average risk adults age 50 to 80
should be offered at least one of the
following colon cancer screening tests:
  - FOBT (if not done in the past 2 years)
  - Sigmoidoscopy (if not done in the past 5
    years)
  - Colonoscopy (if not done in the past 10
    years)
  - Double contrast barium enema (if not done
    in the past 5 years)

```
                         3 3 3              1 1 4 3
             1 2 3 4 5 6 7 8 9    1 2 3 4 5 6 7 8 9   ( 21- 22)
               (8.0, 0.7, A)        (8.0, 0.7, A)
```

Scales: 1 = low validity or feasibility; 9 = high validity or feasibility

	Validity	Feasibility

11. Colonoscopy screening should not be done in average risk patients more frequently than every 5 years provided the previous colonoscopy was negative and procedure note specifies adequate exam.

```
                    3 3 3              1 1 3 4
          1 2 3 4 5 6 7 8 9  1 2 3 4 5 6 7 8 9   ( 23- 24)
            (8.0, 0.7, A)       (8.0, 0.8, A)
```

Scales: 1 = low validity or feasibility; 9 = high validity or feasibility

STAGING

1. Patients who have undergone surgical
resection for colon or rectal cancer should
have documentation in the chart that
colonoscopy or barium enema with
sigmoidoscopy was offered within the
preceding 12 months.

```
        1       4 2 2                    1 3 5
1 2 3 4 5 6 7 8 9   1 2 3 4 5 6 7 8 9  ( 1- 2)
   (7.0, 1.1, A)       (9.0, 0.6, A)
```

TREATMENT

2. Patients diagnosed with a malignant polyp
should be offered a wide surgical resection
within 6 weeks if any of the following are
true:

a. the colonoscopy report states that the
polyp was not completely excised

```
        1 2 6                          1 4 4
1 2 3 4 5 6 7 8 9   1 2 3 4 5 6 7 8 9  ( 3- 4)
   (9.0, 0.4, A)       (8.0, 0.6, A)
```

b. the margins are positive

```
        3 6                            5 4
1 2 3 4 5 6 7 8 9   1 2 3 4 5 6 7 8 9  ( 5- 6)
   (9.0, 0.3, A)       (8.0, 0.4, A)
```

c. lymphatic or venous invasion is present

```
        4 5                            5 4
1 2 3 4 5 6 7 8 9   1 2 3 4 5 6 7 8 9  ( 7- 8)
   (9.0, 0.4, A)       (8.0, 0.4, A)
```

d. histology is grade 3 or poorly
differentiated.

```
      5 4                            5 4
1 2 3 4 5 6 7 8 9   1 2 3 4 5 6 7 8 9  ( 9- 10)
   (8.0, 0.4, A)       (8.0, 0.4, A)
```

3. Patients with a malignant polyp treated
with polypectomy alone should be offered
colonoscopy within 6 months of the
polypectomy.

```
        2 5 2                        2 2 5
1 2 3 4 5 6 7 8 9   1 2 3 4 5 6 7 8 9  ( 11- 12)
   (8.0, 0.4, A)       (9.0, 0.7, A)
```

4. Patients who are diagnosed with colon
cancer and do not have metastatic disease
should be offered a wide resection with
anastamosis within 6 weeks of diagnosis.

```
      5 4                            5 4
1 2 3 4 5 6 7 8 9   1 2 3 4 5 6 7 8 9  ( 13- 14)
   (8.0, 0.4, A)       (8.0, 0.4, A)
```

5. Patients who undergo a wide surgical
resection should have "negative margins"
noted on the most recent final pathology
report or have documentation that they were
offered a repeat resection if they meet
either of the following criteria:

a. Stage I colon cancer

```
      4 5                          1 2 6
1 2 3 4 5 6 7 8 9   1 2 3 4 5 6 7 8 9  ( 15- 16)
   (9.0, 0.4, A)       (9.0, 0.4, A)
```

b. Stage II or III colon cancer that is not
invading into other organs (not a T4
lesion)

```
        1 3 5                        1 1 7
1 2 3 4 5 6 7 8 9   1 2 3 4 5 6 7 8 9  ( 17- 18)
   (9.0, 0.6, A)       (9.0, 0.3, A)
```

6. Patients with Stage III colon cancer who
have undergone a surgical resection should be
offered adjuvant chemotherapy to start within
6 weeks of surgery with a published
5-FU-containing regimen (or be enrolled in a
clinical trial with documentation of informed
consent).

```
        1 3 5                        1 3 5
1 2 3 4 5 6 7 8 9   1 2 3 4 5 6 7 8 9  ( 19- 20)
   (9.0, 0.6, A)       (9.0, 0.6, A)
```

Scales: 1 = low validity or feasibility; 9 = high validity or feasibility

TREATMENT, CONT.

7. Patients who are diagnosed preoperatively
with Stage I rectal cancer should be offered
one of the following surgical resections
within 6 weeks of diagnosis (or be enrolled
in a clinical trial with documentation of
informed consent):

- low anterior resection
- abdominal perineal resection
- full-thickness local excision

	Validity	Feasibility	
	4 5	1 3 5	
	1 2 3 4 5 6 7 8 9	1 2 3 4 5 6 7 8 9	(21- 22)
	(9.0, 0.4, A)	(9.0, 0.6, A)	

8. Patients who are diagnosed with rectal
cancer that appears clinically to be Stage II
or III, should be offered one of the
following surgical resections within 6 weeks
of diagnosis or completion of preoperative
therapy (unless enrolled in a clinical trial
with documentation of informed consent):

- low anterior resection
- abdominal perineal resection

	4 5	4 5	
	1 2 3 4 5 6 7 8 9	1 2 3 4 5 6 7 8 9	(23- 24)
	(9.0, 0.4, A)	(9.0, 0.4, A)	

9. Patients who undergo a wide surgical
resection should have "negative margins"
noted on the most recent final pathology
report or have documentation that they were
offered a repeat resection if they meet
either of the following criteria:

a. Stage I rectal cancer

	4 5	1 3 5	
	1 2 3 4 5 6 7 8 9	1 2 3 4 5 6 7 8 9	(25- 26)
	(9.0, 0.4, A)	(9.0, 0.6, A)	

b. Stage II or III rectal cancer that is
not invading into other organs (not a T4
lesion)

	2 3 4	1 4 4	
	1 2 3 4 5 6 7 8 9	1 2 3 4 5 6 7 8 9	(27- 28)
	(8.0, 0.7, A)	(8.0, 0.6, A)	

10. Patients with Stage II and III rectal
cancer (defined pathologically) who undergo
surgical resection should be offered one of
the following treatments (or be enrolled
in a clinical trial with documentation of
informed consent):

- postoperative radiation therapy of
  45-55 Gy to the pelvis with chemotherapy
  containing 5FU to begin not sooner than 4
  weeks after surgery and not more than 12
  weeks after surgery
- preoperative radiation therapy to the
  pelvis to begin not more than 6 weeks
  after diagnosis and discussion of postoperative therapy
- preoperative radiation therapy with
  chemotherapy containing 5FU to begin not
  more than 6 weeks after diagnosis and
  discussion of postoperative therapy

	1 3 2 3	4 2 3	
	1 2 3 4 5 6 7 8 9	1 2 3 4 5 6 7 8 9	(29- 30)
	(8.0, 0.9, A)	(8.0, 0.8, A)	

11. Patients receiving 5-FU chemotherapy
should have a CBC checked not more than 48
hours prior to the first dose in each cycle.

	4 1 2 1 1	4 1 2 1 1	
	1 2 3 4 5 6 7 8 9	1 2 3 4 5 6 7 8 9	(31- 32)
	(2.0, 1.7, A)	(2.0, 1.8, A)	

Scales: 1 = low validity or feasibility; 9 = high validity or feasibility

TREATMENT, CONT.

12. Patients should not receive 5-FU
chemotherapy if any of the following are
documented in the 2 days prior to initiation
of therapy:

                                         5 1   2 1   4 1 1   2 1

   a. WBC < 2,000 or ANC < 1,500   1 2 3 4 5 6 7 8 9 1 2 3 4 5 6 7 8 9 (33- 34)
                                     (1.0, 2.3, D)   (2.0, 2.6, D)

   b. stomatitis that prevents them from   5 1   1 1 1 4 1 1   1 2
   eating   1 2 3 4 5 6 7 8 9 1 2 3 4 5 6 7 8 9 (35- 36)
                                       (1.0, 2.6, D)   (2.0, 2.8, D)

   c. severe diarrhea (seven or more stools 5 1   1 1 1 4 1 1   1 2
   a day)   1 2 3 4 5 6 7 8 9 1 2 3 4 5 6 7 8 9 (37- 38)
                                       (1.0, 2.6, D)   (2.0, 2.8, D)

FOLLOW-UP

13. Patients with Stages I, II, and III
colorectal cancer should receive a visit with
a physician for a history and physical where
colorectal cancer is addressed in the
assessment and plan at least every 6 months 4   1   1 2 1 3   1 1 1 2 1
for 3 years after initiation of treatment.   1 2 3 4 5 6 7 8 9 1 2 3 4 5 6 7 8 9 (39- 40)
                                       (5.0, 3.1, D)   (6.0, 2.7, D)

14. Patients with Stages I, II, and III
colorectal cancer should receive colonoscopy
or double contrast barium enema within a year
of curative surgery if it did not occur   2 5 2 1 1   2 3 2
within 12 months preoperatively.   1 2 3 4 5 6 7 8 9 1 2 3 4 5 6 7 8 9 (41- 42)
                                       (8.0, 0.4, A)   (8.0, 1.9, A)

15. Patients with Stages I, II, and III
colorectal cancer should receive colonoscopy
or double contrast barium enema within one
year after surgery and, if normal, at least   1 5 3   1 3 5
every five years thereafter.   1 2 3 4 5 6 7 8 9 1 2 3 4 5 6 7 8 9 (43- 44)
                                       (8.0, 0.4, A)   (9.0, 0.6, A)

INDICATOR ADDED AFTER ROUND 1

16. Patients with metastatic colon cancer
should have therapeutic discussed within
three weeks of staging (unless enrolled
in a clinical trial with documentation of   1 4 4   1   3 5
informed consent).   1 2 3 4 5 6 7 8 9 1 2 3 4 5 6 7 8 9 (45- 46)
                                       (8.0, 0.6, A)   (9.0, 0.7, A)

Scales: 1 = low validity or feasibility; 9 = high validity or feasibility

SCREENING AND PREVENTION

| | Validity | Feasibility | |

1. HIV+ patients should be offered PCP prophylaxis within one month of meeting any of the following conditions:

a. CD4 count dropping below 200
```
          1 8                       3 6
1 2 3 4 5 6 7 8 9     1 2 3 4 5 6 7 8 9    ( 1- 2)
  (9.0, 0.1, A)         (9.0, 0.3, A)
```

b. Thrush
```
2 1 2  1 1    2        2      1 1 1 2 2
1 2 3 4 5 6 7 8 9     1 2 3 4 5 6 7 8 9    ( 3- 4)
  (3.0, 2.2, I)         (7.0, 2.3, I)
```

c. Completion of active treatment of PCP
```
            2 7                     3 6
1 2 3 4 5 6 7 8 9     1 2 3 4 5 6 7 8 9    ( 5- 6)
  (9.0, 0.2, A)         (9.0, 0.3, A)
```

d. CD4 below 15%
```
        1 1 1 6                     3 6
1 2 3 4 5 6 7 8 9     1 2 3 4 5 6 7 8 9    ( 7- 8)
  (9.0, 0.7, A)         (9.0, 0.3, A)
```

2. HIV+ patients who do not have active TB and who have not ever previously received TB prophylaxis should be offered TB prophylaxis within one month of meeting any of following conditions:

a. Current PPD > 5 mm
```
        1 3 5                     1 3 5
1 2 3 4 5 6 7 8 9     1 2 3 4 5 6 7 8 9    ( 9- 10)
  (9.0, 0.6, A)         (9.0, 0.6, A)
```

b. Provider noting that patient has had PPD > 5 mm administered at anytime since HIV diagnosis
```
      2 4 3             1   1 3 1 3
1 2 3 4 5 6 7 8 9     1 2 3 4 5 6 7 8 9    ( 11- 12)
  (8.0, 0.6, A)         (7.0, 1.2, A)
```

c. Contact with person with active TB
```
2   1   1   1 2 2     2   1 2 1 3
1 2 3 4 5 6 7 8 9     1 2 3 4 5 6 7 8 9    ( 13- 14)
  (7.0, 2.7, D)         (4.0, 1.6, I)
```

3. HIV+ patients who do not have active toxoplasmosis should be offered toxoplasmosis prophylaxis within one month of meeting either of the following conditions:

- Toxo IgG positive and CD4 count dropping below 100
- Completion of therapy for active toxoplasmosis
```
          3   6                   2 2 5
1 2 3 4 5 6 7 8 9     1 2 3 4 5 6 7 8 9    ( 15- 16)
  (9.0, 0.7, A)         (9.0, 0.7, A)
```

4. HIV+ patients should have toxoplasmosis serology documented.
```
        4 1 4                     3 4 2
1 2 3 4 5 6 7 8 9     1 2 3 4 5 6 7 8 9    ( 17- 18)
  (8.0, 0.9, A)         (8.0, 0.6, A)
```

5. HIV+ patients should be offered MAC prophylaxis within one month of a CD4 count dropping below 50.
```
          2 2 5                   3 2 4
1 2 3 4 5 6 7 8 9     1 2 3 4 5 6 7 8 9    ( 19- 20)
  (9.0, 0.7, A)         (8.0, 0.8, A)
```

6. HIV+ patients with a lowest recorded CD4 > 200 should have a documented pneumovax.
```
      1 3 3 2         1       1 5   2
1 2 3 4 5 6 7 8 9     1 2 3 4 5 6 7 8 9    ( 21- 22)
  (8.0, 0.8, A)         (7.0, 1.1, A)
```

7. HIV+ patients with a lowest recorded CD4 count of less than 100 should have had a yearly dilated fundoscopic exam.
```
        4 2 3               1 2 3 3
1 2 3 4 5 6 7 8 9     1 2 3 4 5 6 7 8 9    ( 23- 24)
  (8.0, 0.8, A)         (8.0, 0.8, A)
```

8. HIV+ patients should have a VDRL or RPR documented in the chart.
```
        3 2 4                     2 3 4
1 2 3 4 5 6 7 8 9     1 2 3 4 5 6 7 8 9    ( 25- 26)
  (8.0, 0.8, A)         (8.0, 0.7, A)
```

9. Sexually active HIV+ patients should be offered a VDRL/RPR annually.
```
7     1     1         5 1 1   2
1 2 3 4 5 6 7 8 9     1 2 3 4 5 6 7 8 9    ( 27- 28)
  (1.0, 1.0, A)         (1.0, 1.2, A)
```

Scales: 1 = low validity or feasibility; 9 = high validity or feasibility

DIAGNOSIS

10. The following tests should be obtained
within one month of initial diagnosis of HIV
infection:

                                                      2 3 4   2 2 5
  a. CBC   1 2 3 4 5 6 7 8 9   1 2 3 4 5 6 7 8 9   (29- 30)
                                           (8.0, 0.7, A)   (9.0, 0.7, A)
                                                      2 2 5   2 1 6
  b. HIV RNA (viral load)   1 2 3 4 5 6 7 8 9   1 2 3 4 5 6 7 8 9   (31- 32)
                                           (9.0, 0.7, A)   (9.0, 0.6, A)
                                                      2 1 6   2 1 6
  c. CD4   1 2 3 4 5 6 7 8 9   1 2 3 4 5 6 7 8 9   (33- 34)
                                           (9.0, 0.6, A)   (9.0, 0.6, A)

11. HIV+ patients with CD4 counts > 300
should be offered the following tests every
6 months:

                                                      2 2 5   1 2 6
  a. CD4 count or percentage   1 2 3 4 5 6 7 8 9   1 2 3 4 5 6 7 8 9   (35- 36)
                                           (9.0, 0.7, A)   (9.0, 0.4, A)
                                                      2 2 5   1 2 6
  b. HIV RNA (viral load)   1 2 3 4 5 6 7 8 9   1 2 3 4 5 6 7 8 9   (37- 38)
                                           (9.0, 0.7, A)   (9.0, 0.4, A)

12. HIV+ patients with detectable viral
loads should be offered the following tests
within 3 months:

                                          1 1 1   1 2 1 2   1   2   1   2   3
  a. CD4 count or percentage   1 2 3 4 5 6 7 8 9   1 2 3 4 5 6 7 8 9   (39- 40)
                                           (6.0, 2.0, D)   (7.0, 2.4, D)
                                                      2 2 5   4 5
  b. HIV RNA (viral load)   1 2 3 4 5 6 7 8 9   1 2 3 4 5 6 7 8 9   (41- 42)
                                           (9.0, 0.7, A)   (9.0, 0.9, A)

13. HIV+ patients on antiretroviral therapy
should have been offered the following tests
within the past 4 months:

                                                      2 3 4   2 3 4
  a. CD4 count or percentage   1 2 3 4 5 6 7 8 9   1 2 3 4 5 6 7 8 9   (43- 44)
                                           (8.0, 0.7, A)   (8.0, 0.7, A)
                                                      1 3 5   1   1 2 5
  b. HIV RNA (viral load)   1 2 3 4 5 6 7 8 9   1 2 3 4 5 6 7 8 9   (45- 46)
                                           (9.0, 0.6, A)   (9.0, 1.0, A)
                                                        3 6   1 3 5
  c. CBC   1 2 3 4 5 6 7 8 9   1 2 3 4 5 6 7 8 9   (47- 48)
                                           (9.0, 0.3, A)   (9.0, 0.6, A)

Scales: 1 = low validity or feasibility; 9 = high validity or feasibility

	Validity	Feasibility

TREATMENT

14. HIV+ patients should receive adequate antiretroviral treatment within one month of any of the following conditions being met (or be enrolled in a clinical trial with documentation of informed consent):

a. CD4 >= 500 and viral load >30k

```
              2 2 5                    2 3 4
1 2 3 4 5 6 7 8 9    1 2 3 4 5 6 7 8 9   ( 49- 50)
   (9.0, 0.7, A)        (8.0, 0.7, A)
```

b. CD4 350-499 and viral load >10k

```
                4 5                      1 4 4
1 2 3 4 5 6 7 8 9    1 2 3 4 5 6 7 8 9   ( 51- 52)
   (9.0, 0.4, A)        (8.0, 0.6, A)
```

c. CD4 < 350

```
              1 4 4                      1 4 4
1 2 3 4 5 6 7 8 9    1 2 3 4 5 6 7 8 9   ( 53- 54)
   (8.0, 0.6, A)        (8.0, 0.6, A)
```

d. Any AIDS-defining condition

```
                4 5                      1 3 5
1 2 3 4 5 6 7 8 9    1 2 3 4 5 6 7 8 9   ( 55- 56)
   (9.0, 0.4, A)        (9.0, 0.6, A)
```

e. thrush

```
     1     2 2 2 2   1     2   3 3
1 2 3 4 5 6 7 8 9    1 2 3 4 5 6 7 8 9   ( 57- 58)
   (7.0, 1.3, I)        (8.0, 1.4, I)
```

15. Protease inhibitors should not be prescribed concurrently with astemizole, terfenadine, rifampin or cisapride.

```
            1 5 3      1       3 2 3
1 2 3 4 5 6 7 8 9    1 2 3 4 5 6 7 8 9   ( 59- 60)
   (8.0, 0.4, A)        (8.0, 1.1, A)
```

FOLLOW-UP

16. HIV+ patients should be offered viral load measurement within two months of initiation or change in antiretroviral treatment.

```
            5 1 3                  2 3 4
1 2 3 4 5 6 7 8 9    1 2 3 4 5 6 7 8 9   ( 61- 62)
   (7.0, 0.8, A)        (8.0, 0.7, A)
```

INDICATORS ADDED AFTER ROUND 1

17. HIV+ patients started on protease inhibitors should have documented counseling regarding compliance with therapy within 1 month of the start of therapy.

```
            5 4                   1 4 3 1
1 2 3 4 5 6 7 8 9    1 2 3 4 5 6 7 8 9   ( 63- 64)
   (8.0, 0.4, A)        (7.0, 0.7, A)
```

18. HIV+ patients should be counseled regarding high risk behavior:

a. at the time of HIV diagnosis

```
            2 3 4                      4 2 3
1 2 3 4 5 6 7 8 9    1 2 3 4 5 6 7 8 9   ( 65- 66)
   (8.0, 0.7, A)        (8.0, 0.8, A)
```

b. within 1 month of presentation with an initial infection of STD

```
            5 2 2    1     2 1 2 1 2
1 2 3 4 5 6 7 8 9    1 2 3 4 5 6 7 8 9   ( 67- 68)
   (7.0, 0.7, A)        (7.0, 1.7, I)
```

Scales: 1 = low validity or feasibility; 9 = high validity or feasibility

DIAGNOSIS

1. Patients without a prior diagnosis of
metastatic cancer with a solitary mass
(>= 3 cm) on chest x-ray or CT scan of
the chest should have a tissue or cytologic
diagnosis of pathologic process documented
in the chart within 2 months of the
radiological study unless contraindicated.

```
            1    4 2 2  1              1 4 1 2
1 2 3 4 5 6 7 8 9  1 2 3 4 5 6 7 8 9  ( 1- 2)
   (7.0, 0.9, A)       (7.0, 1.3, A)
```

2. Patients without a prior diagnosis of
cancer (except non-melanoma skin cancer) with
a solitary nodule (< 3 cm) on chest x-ray or
CT scan of the chest should have one of the
following documented in the chart within 2
months of the radiological study:

- Report of chest x-ray or CT scan of the
  chest from at least 2 years prior to the
  index study which shows a nodule of the
  same size in the same location
- Chest x-ray or CT scan report describes
  the nodule has having central, diffuse,
  speckled, or laminar calcifications
- Chest CT scan report states that the
  density of the nodule is > 160 Hounsfield
  units
- Chest CT with multiple nodules
- Sputum cytology, bronchoscopic washing,
  or bronchoscopic brushing diagnostic of
  cancer
- Cytology report from a fine needle
  aspiration of the mass
- Pathology report from lymph node biopsy
  that is diagnostic of cancer
- Pathology report from biopsy of nodule
- Operative report indicating surgical
  resection of the mass.

```
 1   2      6    1    2     2 3 1
1 2 3 4 5 6 7 8 9  1 2 3 4 5 6 7 8 9  ( 3- 4)
   (7.0, 1.2, I)       (7.0, 1.9, I)
```

Scales: 1 = low validity or feasibility; 9 = high validity or feasibility

TREATMENT

3. Patients with non-small cell lung cancer should have both of the following not more than 3 months prior to lung resection:

a. Pulmonary function assessment with either pulmonary function tests (FEV1, maximum ventilatory volume) or a quantitative ventilation scan or a quantitative perfusion scan

```
                5 4                   3 6
1 2 3 4 5 6 7 8 9   1 2 3 4 5 6 7 8 9   ( 5-  6)
   (8.0, 0.4, A)       (9.0, 0.3, A)
```

b. EKG

```
                1 4 4                 3 6
1 2 3 4 5 6 7 8 9   1 2 3 4 5 6 7 8 9   ( 7-  8)
   (8.0, 0.6, A)       (9.0, 0.3, A)
```

4. Patients with Stage I and II non-small cell lung cancer should be offered a lung resection (pneumonectomy, lobectomy, or wedge resection) within 6 weeks of diagnosis unless contraindicated.

```
                1 4 4                 1 4 4
1 2 3 4 5 6 7 8 9   1 2 3 4 5 6 7 8 9   ( 9- 10)
   (8.0, 0.6, A)       (8.0, 0.6, A)
```

5. Patients with Stage I or II non-small cell lung cancer who do not undergo a lung resection should be offered radiation therapy to the chest (>=5000 cGy) within 6 weeks of diagnosis.

```
                4 5                 3 2 4
1 2 3 4 5 6 7 8 9   1 2 3 4 5 6 7 8 9   ( 11- 12)
   (8.0, 0.4, A)       (8.0, 0.8, A)
```

6. Patients with Stage III non-small cell lung cancer with good performance status should be offered at least one of the following within 6 weeks of diagnosis (unless contraindicated or enrolled in a clinical trial with documentation of informed consent):

- thoracotomy with surgical resection of the tumor
- radiation therapy to the thorax with chemotherapy

```
              6 1 2         1       4 1 3
1 2 3 4 5 6 7 8 9   1 2 3 4 5 6 7 8 9   ( 13- 14)
   (7.0, 0.6, A)       (7.0, 1.2, A)
```

7. Patients with Stage IV non-small cell lung cancer and good performance status should have chemotherapy discussed within 6 weeks of diagnosis (or be enrolled in a clinical trial with documentation of informed consent).

```
                4 5           1   2 3 3
1 2 3 4 5 6 7 8 9   1 2 3 4 5 6 7 8 9   ( 15- 16)
   (8.0, 0.4, A)       (7.0, 0.9, I)
```

Scales: 1 = low validity or feasibility; 9 = high validity or feasibility

TREATMENT, CONT.

8. Patients with non-small cell lung cancer
who have first metastases on MRI or CT of the
brain should be offered one of the following
treatments within 1 week of the MRI or CT
(or be enrolled in a clinical trial with
documentation of informed consent):

- radiation therapy to the brain
- surgical resection of the metastasis
- stereotactic radiosurgery

```
                        1   4 4                  2 4 3
              1 2 3 4 5 6 7 8 9    1 2 3 4 5 6 7 8 9    ( 17- 18)
                (8.0, 0.7, A)        (8.0, 0.6, A)
```

9. Patients with limited small cell lung
cancer should be offered combined modality
therapy with radiation therapy (>= 5,000 cGy)
and chemotherapy within 2 weeks of diagnosis
(or be enrolled in a clinical trial with
documentation of informed consent).

```
                      1 3 5                      5 4
              1 2 3 4 5 6 7 8 9    1 2 3 4 5 6 7 8 9    ( 19- 20)
                (9.0, 0.6, A)        (8.0, 0.4, A)
```

10. Patients with extensive small cell lung
cancer should be offered chemotherapy within
2 weeks of diagnosis.

```
                        4 5                    1 4 4
              1 2 3 4 5 6 7 8 9    1 2 3 4 5 6 7 8 9    ( 21- 22)
                (9.0, 0.4, A)        (8.0, 0.6, A)
```

11. Patients with small cell lung cancer who
have first metastases on MRI or CT of the
brain should be offered either of the
following within 1 week of diagnosis of
brain metastases (unless they have received
both previously):

- chemotherapy
- radiation therapy to the brain

```
                      3 2 4                    1 5 3
              1 2 3 4 5 6 7 8 9    1 2 3 4 5 6 7 8 9    ( 23- 24)
                (8.0, 0.8, A)        (8.0, 0.4, A)
```

12. Patients with small cell lung cancer who
have bone pain and a corresponding positive
radiographic study should be offered either
of the following within 1 week of presenting
with the complaint of pain (unless they have
received both previously):

- chemotherapy
- radiation therapy to the region

```
              3 2           2 1 1  1 1            3 2 2
              1 2 3 4 5 6 7 8 9    1 2 3 4 5 6 7 8 9    ( 25- 26)
                (2.0, 2.9, D)        (7.0, 1.9, A)
```

Scales: 1 = low validity or feasibility; 9 = high validity or feasibility

NOTE: There are no recommended indicators for
this chapter.

	Validity	Feasibility

DIAGNOSIS

1. Men without any previously known diagnosis of cancer who have an x-ray or radionuclide bone scan with blastic or lytic lesions, or with a notation that the findings are consistent with metastases, should be offered both of the following within the 12 months prior to or 3 weeks following the date of the x-ray or bone scan:

```
                            6           2 1      4 1 1      1 1   1
   a. digital rectal exam   1 2 3 4 5 6 7 8 9  1 2 3 4 5 6 7 8 9  ( 1-  2)
                              (1.0, 2.1, D)       (2.0, 2.3, I)
                            6           1 1 1 5   1        1 1   1
   b. PSA                   1 2 3 4 5 6 7 8 9  1 2 3 4 5 6 7 8 9  ( 3-  4)
                              (1.0, 2.3, D)       (1.0, 2.3, I)
```

2. Men with a new diagnosis of prostate cancer, who have not had a serum PSA in the prior 3 months, should have serum PSA checked within 1 month after diagnosis or prior to any treatment, whichever comes first.

```
                                      1 4 4                2 7
                            1 2 3 4 5 6 7 8 9  1 2 3 4 5 6 7 8 9  ( 5-  6)
                              (8.0, 0.6, A)       (9.0, 0.2, A)
```

3. Men with a new diagnosis of prostate cancer who have a PSA > 10mg/ml should be offered a radionuclide bone scan within 1 month or prior to initiation of any treatment, whichever comes first.

```
                                      1 4 4                4 5
                            1 2 3 4 5 6 7 8 9  1 2 3 4 5 6 7 8 9  ( 7-  8)
                              (8.0, 0.6, A)       (9.0, 0.4, A)
```

TREATMENT

4. "O" Men over 60 with minimal prostate cancer (Stage O/A1) should not be offered any of the following treatments:

```
                            1           1 3 4 1              4 4
   a. bilateral orchiectomy 1 2 3 4 5 6 7 8 9  1 2 3 4 5 6 7 8 9  ( 9- 10)
                              (8.0, 1.3, A)       (8.0, 1.2, A)
                            1               4 4 1            4 4
   b. LHRH analogue         1 2 3 4 5 6 7 8 9  1 2 3 4 5 6 7 8 9  (11- 12)
                              (8.0, 1.2, A)       (8.0, 1.2, A)
                            1               4 4 1            4 4
   c. antiandrogen          1 2 3 4 5 6 7 8 9  1 2 3 4 5 6 7 8 9  (13- 14)
                              (8.0, 1.2, A)       (8.0, 1.2, A)
                            2 1     1     2 3 1     1      1 3 3
   d. radical prostatectomy 1 2 3 4 5 6 7 8 9  1 2 3 4 5 6 7 8 9  (15- 16)
                              (8.0, 2.9, D)       (8.0, 1.7, A)
                            2 1     1     2 3 1     1      1 3 3
   e. radiation therapy     1 2 3 4 5 6 7 8 9  1 2 3 4 5 6 7 8 9  (17- 18)
                              (8.0, 2.9, D)       (8.0, 1.7, A)
```

4. "X" Patients with prostate cancer (Stage T1C with Gleason <= 4 and PSA <= 10) should not be offered any of the following treatments:

```
                                    2 3 4              1 4 4
   a. bilateral orchiectomy 1 2 3 4 5 6 7 8 9  1 2 3 4 5 6 7 8 9  (19- 20)
                              (8.0, 0.7, A)       (8.0, 0.6, A)
                                    2 3 4              1 4 4
   b. LHRH analogue         1 2 3 4 5 6 7 8 9  1 2 3 4 5 6 7 8 9  (21- 22)
                              (8.0, 0.7, A)       (8.0, 0.6, A)
                                    2 3 4              1 4 4
   c. antiandrogen          1 2 3 4 5 6 7 8 9  1 2 3 4 5 6 7 8 9  (23- 24)
                              (8.0, 0.7, A)       (8.0, 0.6, A)
```

Scales: 1 = low validity or feasibility; 9 = high validity or feasibility

TREATMENT, CONT.

5. Men under 65 with localized prostate
cancer(Stage I or II/A2 or B) and a Gleason
score <= 6 should have all of the following
treatment options discussed within 3 months
of diagnosis (unless contraindicated or
enrolled in a clinical trial with
documentation of informed consent):

   - radiation therapy   2 5 2   1 1 4 3
   - prostatectomy   1 2 3 4 5 6 7 8 9 1 2 3 4 5 6 7 8 9 (25- 26)
   - watchful waiting   (8.0, 0.4, A)   (8.0, 0.7, A)

6. Men with metastatic prostate cancer
(Stage IV/D) should be offered at least one
of the following androgen blockade treatments
within three months of staging:

   - bilateral orchiectomy
   - LHRH analogue with or without   6 3   5 4
     antiandrogen   1 2 3 4 5 6 7 8 9 1 2 3 4 5 6 7 8 9 (27- 28)
                     (8.0, 0.3, A)   (8.0, 0.4, A)

7. Men who undergo orchiectomy for the
treatment of prostate cancer should have
documented that they were offered treatment
with an LHRH analogue (with or without
antiandrogen) within 12 months prior to   1 2 2 4   3 3 3
surgery.   1 2 3 4 5 6 7 8 9 1 2 3 4 5 6 7 8 9 (29- 30)
                     (8.0, 0.9, A)   (8.0, 0.7, A)

8. Metastatic prostate cancer patients who
present with acute back pain with
radiculopathy should have documentation
within 24 hours of presentation of one of
the following:

   - a CT scan of the spine without blastic
     or lytic lesions or compression fractures
   - a CT myelogram   1   2 3 3   5 4
   - an MRI of the spine   1 2 3 4 5 6 7 8 9 1 2 3 4 5 6 7 8 9 (31- 32)
                     (8.0, 1.0, A)   (8.0, 0.4, A)

9. Prostate cancer patients with evidence of
cord compression from tumor on MRI scan of
the spine or CT myelogram should be offered
one of the following within 24 hours of the
radiologic study:

   - radiation therapy to the spine at a total
     dose between 3000cGy and 4500cGy over 2-4
     weeks   1 3 5   1   1 2 5
   - decompressive laminectomy 1 2 3 4 5 6 7 8 9 1 2 3 4 5 6 7 8 9 (33- 34)
                     (9.0, 0.6, A)   (9.0, 1.1, A)

10. Prostate cancer patients with evidence
of cord compression from tumor on MRI scan of
the spine or CT myelogram should be offered
at least 4 mg dexamethazone IV prior to the
radiologic study or within 1 hour of its
completion, followed by dexamethasone   2 2 4   1   1 2 4
4mg IV or PO q 6 hours for at least 72 hours. 1 2 3 4 5 6 7 8 9 1 2 3 4 5 6 7 8 9 (35- 36)
                     (8.5, 0.8, A)   (8.5, 1.5, A)

Scales: 1 = low validity or feasibility; 9 = high validity or feasibility

INDICATORS ADDED AFTER ROUND 1

11. Men under age 75 with localized prostate
cancer (Stage I or II/A2 or B) and a Gleason
score >= 7 should be offered both of the
following treatment options within 3 months
of diagnosis (unless contraindicated or
enrolled in a clinical trial with
documentation of informed consent):

- radiation therapy	4 4 1	3 3 3
- radical prostatectomy	1 2 3 4 5 6 7 8 9	1 2 3 4 5 6 7 8 9 (37- 38)
	(8.0, 0.6, A)	(8.0, 0.7, A)

12. Men with prostate cancer who present
with acute back pain should have the presence
or absence of all of the following elicited
on the day of presentation:

a. bladder dysfunction	3 6	4 1 4
	1 2 3 4 5 6 7 8 9	1 2 3 4 5 6 7 8 9 (39- 40)
	(9.0, 0.3, A)	(8.0, 0.9, A)
b. bowel dysfunction	3 6	4 1 4
	1 2 3 4 5 6 7 8 9	1 2 3 4 5 6 7 8 9 (41- 42)
	(9.0, 0.3, A)	(8.0, 0.9, A)
c. weakness or radicular symptoms	3 6	1 3 1 4
	1 2 3 4 5 6 7 8 9	1 2 3 4 5 6 7 8 9 (43- 44)
	(9.0, 0.3, A)	(8.0, 1.0, A)
d. sensory loss	1 2 6	1 3 2 3
	1 2 3 4 5 6 7 8 9	1 2 3 4 5 6 7 8 9 (45- 46)
	(9.0, 1.1, A)	(8.0, 0.9, A)

| | Validity | Feasibility |

PRIMARY PREVENTION

1. When a patient is noted to have a sunburn, the chart should document counseling regarding avoidance of midday sun, use of protective clothing, and/or use of sunscreens.

```
1     1   2 3 2     4 1 3   1
1 2 3 4 5 6 7 8 9   1 2 3 4 5 6 7 8 9   ( 1- 2)
   (7.0, 1.4, I)       (2.0, 1.1, A)
```

2. Patients who have evidence of aktinic keratosis or solar keratosis (AK), should be counseled regarding avoidance of midday sun, use of protective clothing, and/or use of sunscreens within 1 year before or after diagnosis.

```
              4 4 1       1     5 3
1 2 3 4 5 6 7 8 9   1 2 3 4 5 6 7 8 9   ( 3- 4)
   (8.0, 0.6, A)       (7.0, 0.7, A)
```

3. All patients noted to have strong skin cancer risk factors should be instructed in midday sun avoidance, use of protective clothing, and/or use of sunscreens within 1 year before or after note of high risk.

```
        1   5 3     3 2 1 1   2
1 2 3 4 5 6 7 8 9   1 2 3 4 5 6 7 8 9   ( 5- 6)
   (7.0, 0.6, A)       (3.0, 1.6, I)
```

SECONDARY PREVENTION/SKIN SELF-EXAM

4. All patients noted to have strong skin cancer risk factors should be instructed in skin self-examination within 1 year before or after note of high risk.

```
1   1 3 4       2 1   3 1 2
1 2 3 4 5 6 7 8 9   1 2 3 4 5 6 7 8 9   ( 7- 8)
   (5.0, 0.9, A)       (5.0, 1.4, I)
```

5. All patients with a personal history of melanoma should be counseled to do skin self-examination within 1 year before or after the history is documented.

```
              7   2           7 1 1
1 2 3 4 5 6 7 8 9   1 2 3 4 5 6 7 8 9   ( 9- 10)
   (7.0, 0.4, A)       (7.0, 0.3, A)
```

SECONDARY PREVENTION/CLINICIAN SCREENING

6. Patients with a history of NMSC or multiple AKs in the past 5 years should have a skin exam documented in the past 12 months.

```
              2 5 2           3 4 2
1 2 3 4 5 6 7 8 9   1 2 3 4 5 6 7 8 9   ( 11- 12)
   (8.0, 0.4, A)       (8.0, 0.6, A)
```

8. All patients newly diagnosed with melanoma should be advised to have family members undergo a screening skin exam.

```
1         4 4         2 3 2 2
1 2 3 4 5 6 7 8 9   1 2 3 4 5 6 7 8 9   ( 13- 14)
   (6.0, 1.0, I)       (6.0, 0.9, I)
```

9. "O" All patients with a documented family history of melanoma in a first degree relative should have a screening skin exam at least once in the year preceding or subsequent to documentation.

```
1 2     2 4         1 1 2 5
1 2 3 4 5 6 7 8 9   1 2 3 4 5 6 7 8 9   ( 15- 16)
   (6.0, 1.6, D)       (7.0, 0.8, I)
```

9. "X" All patients with a documented personal history of melanoma in a first degree relative should have a screening skin exam at least once in the year preceding or subsequent to documentation.

```
              3 1 5         2 3 4
1 2 3 4 5 6 7 8 9   1 2 3 4 5 6 7 8 9   ( 17- 18)
   (9.0, 0.8, A)       (8.0, 0.7, A)
```

Scales: 1 = low validity or feasibility; 9 = high validity or feasibility

INDICATORS ADDED AFTER ROUND 1

1. Patients with metastatic cancer to bone should have the presence or absence of pain noted at least every 6 months.

```
                  3 4 2                      6 1 2
          1 2 3 4 5 6 7 8 9    1 2 3 4 5 6 7 8 9    ( 1- 2)
             (8.0, 0.6, A)        (7.0, 0.6, A)
```

2. Cancer patients whose pain is uncontrolled should be offered a change in pain management within 24 hours of the pain complaint.

```
                  1 4 4                    1 1 1 4 2
          1 2 3 4 5 6 7 8 9    1 2 3 4 5 6 7 8 9    ( 3- 4)
             (8.0, 0.6, A)        (8.0, 0.9, A)
```

3. Patients with painful bony metastases, who are noted to be unresponsive to or intolerant of narcotic analgesia, should be offered one of the following within one week of the notation of pain:

  - radiation therapy to the sites of pain
  - radioactive strontium therapy

```
          6 1   1     1      4 1     1 1       2
          1 2 3 4 5 6 7 8 9    1 2 3 4 5 6 7 8 9    ( 5- 6)
             (1.0, 1.1, A)        (2.0, 2.8, I)
```

4. Patients receiving emetogenic chemotherapy should be offered concurrent potent antiemetic therapy (e.g. 5HT blockade).

```
                  4 2 3                    1 1 1 3 3
          1 2 3 4 5 6 7 8 9    1 2 3 4 5 6 7 8 9    ( 7- 8)
             (8.0, 0.8, A)        (8.0, 1.0, A)
```

Scales: 1 = low validity or feasibility; 9 = high validity or feasibility

APPENDIX B: CROSSWALK TABLE OF ORIGINAL AND FINAL INDICATORS

Chapter 1 - Breast Cancer Screening

Original Indicator Proposed by Staff		Indicator Voted on by Panel	Comments/Disposition
Screening			
1. Women aged 52 to 69 should have had a screening mammography performed in the past 2 years.	1.	Women aged **50 to 70** should have had a screening mammography performed in the past **at least every 2 years.**	MODIFIED: Age was modified to reflect the earliest required mammography, rather than age at time of record review. Panelists also wanted to emphasize "every" 2 years. **ACCEPTED AS MODIFIED**
	-- (2)	**Women aged 50-70 should have a clinical breast exam of both breasts at least every two years.**	**PROPOSED BUT DROPPED BY Q2 PANEL** due to **low validity score.** The evidence linking exams to improved outcomes is poor.

257

Chapter 2 - Breast Cancer Diagnosis And Treatment

	Original Indicator Proposed by Staff		Indicator Voted on by Panel	Comments/Disposition
	Diagnosis			
1.	If a palpable breast mass has been detected, at least one of the following procedures should be completed within 3 months: • Fine needle aspiration; • Mammography; • Ultrasound; • Biopsy; • Follow-up visit.	1.	If a palpable breast mass has been detected, at least one of the following procedures should be completed within 3 months: • Fine needle aspiration; • Mammography; • Ultrasound; • Biopsy; • Follow-up visit.	**INCLUDED BASED ON Q1 PANEL RATING**
2.	If a breast mass has been detected on two separate occasions, then either a biopsy, FNA or ultrasound should be performed within 3 months of the second visit.	2.	If a breast mass has been detected on two separate occasions, then either a biopsy, FNA or ultrasound should be performed within 3 months of the second visit.	**INCLUDED BASED ON Q1 PANEL RATING**
3.	A biopsy or FNA should be performed within 6 weeks of either of the following circumstances: a. mammography suggests malignancy; b. persistent palpable mass is not cystic on ultrasound.	3. a. b.	A biopsy or FNA should be performed within 6 weeks of either of the following circumstances: a. mammography suggests malignancy; b. persistent palpable mass is not cystic on ultrasound.	**INCLUDED BASED ON Q1 PANEL RATING**
4.	A biopsy should be performed within 6 weeks if FNA cannot rule out malignancy.	4.	A biopsy should be performed within 6 weeks if FNA cannot rule out malignancy.	**INCLUDED BASED ON Q1 PANEL RATING**
	Treatment			
5.	Women with stage I or stage II breast cancer should be offered a choice of modified radical mastectomy or breast-conserving surgery, unless contraindications to breast- conserving surgery are present.	5.	Women with stage I or stage II breast cancer should be offered a choice of modified radical mastectomy or breast-conserving surgery, unless contraindications to breast-conserving surgery are present.	**ACCEPTED**
6.	Women treated with breast conserving surgery should begin radiation therapy within 6 weeks of completing either of the following (unless wound complications prevent the initiation of treatment): • last surgical procedure on the breast (including reconstructive surgery); or • chemotherapy, if patient receives adjuvant chemotherapy.	6.	Women treated with breast conserving surgery should begin radiation therapy within 6 weeks of completing either of the following (unless wound complications prevent the initiation of treatment): • last surgical procedure on the breast (including reconstructive surgery **that occurs within 6 weeks of primary resection**) • chemotherapy, if patient receives adjuvant chemotherapy	**MODIFIED:** Panelists felt that radiation therapy should not be delayed until after reconstructive surgery if the surgery occurred more than 6 weeks after the primary resection. **ACCEPTED AS MODIFIED**

258

Original Indicator Proposed by Staff		Indicator Voted on by Panel	Comments/Disposition
Treatment			
7. Women with node-positive breast cancer should be treated with adjuvant systemic therapy to include one of the following: • Combination chemotherapy (more than one agent, lasting for at least 2 months); • Tamoxifen (20mg/d for at least 2 years).	7.	Women with node-positive invasive breast cancer **that is node-positive, or node-negative and primary tumor >= 1 cm,** should be treated with adjuvant systemic therapy to include **at least** one of the following: • Combination chemotherapy (more than one agent, lasting for at least 2 months); • Tamoxifen (20mg/d for at least 2 years).	MODIFIED: Panelists wanted to exclude carcinoma-in-situ, and felt that node-negative breast cancers >= 1 cm should also receive chemotherapy. **ACCEPTED AS MODIFIED**
	8. (11)	**Women with metastatic breast cancer should be offered one of the following treatments within 6 weeks of the identification of metastases:** • **Hormonal therapy;** • **Chemotherapy;** • **Enrollment in a clinical trial with documentation of informed consent.**	**PROPOSED AND ACCEPTED BY Q2 PANEL.** Panelists felt that it is important to have an indicator on metastatic breast cancer treatment.
Follow-up			
8. Women with a history of breast cancer should have a yearly mammography.	9.	Women with a history of breast cancer should have a yearly mammography.	ACCEPTED
9. Women diagnosed with breast cancer in the past 5 years should have a clinical breast exam in the past 6 months.	10.	Women diagnosed with breast cancer in the past 5 years should have a clinical breast exam at least once a year ~~in the past 6 months.~~	MODIFIED: Panelists felt that a yearly clinical breast exam is sufficient. **ACCEPTED AS MODIFIED**
10. Women diagnosed with breast cancer more than 5 years ago should have a clinical breast exam in the past year.	11.	Women diagnosed with breast cancer more than 5 years ago should have a clinical breast exam **at least once a year.**	MODIFIED: Panelists wanted to clarify that this is a minimum annual requirement. **ACCEPTED AS MODIFIED**

Chapter 3 - Cervical Cancer Screening

	Original Indicator Proposed by Staff		Indicator Voted on by Panel	Comments/Disposition
	Screening			
1.	The medical record should contain the date and result of the last Pap smear.	1.	The medical record should contain the date and result of the last Pap smear.	INCLUDED BASED ON Q1 PANEL RATING
2.	Women who have not had a Pap smear within the last 3 years should have one performed (unless never sexually active with men or have had a hysterectomy for benign indications).	2.	Women who have not had a Pap smear within the last 3 years should have one performed (unless never sexually active with men or have had a hysterectomy for benign indications).	INCLUDED BASED ON Q1 PANEL RATING
3.	Women who have not had 3 consecutive normal smears and who have not had a Pap smear within the last year should have one performed.	3.	Women who have not had 3 consecutive normal smears and who have not had a Pap smear within the last year should have one performed.	INCLUDED BASED ON Q1 PANEL RATING
4.	Women with a history of cervical dysplasia or carcinoma-in-situ who have not had a Pap smear within the last year should have one performed.	4.	Women with a history of cervical dysplasia, ~~or~~ carcinoma-in-situ **or HIV infection** who have not had a Pap smear within the last year should have one performed.	MODIFIED: Panelists wanted to include HIV positive women who are at high risk for cervical dysplasia. **ACCEPTED AS MODIFIED**
5.	Women with a severely abnormal Pap smear should have colposcopy performed within 3 months of the Pap smear date.	5.	Women with a severely abnormal Pap smear should have colposcopy performed within 3 months of the Pap smear date.	INCLUDED BASED ON Q1 PANEL RATING
6.	If a woman has a Pap smear that shows a low grade lesion (ASCUS or LGSIL), then one of the following should occur within 6 months of the initial Pap: 1) repeat Pap smear; or 2) colposcopy.	6.	If a woman has a Pap smear that shows a low grade lesion (ASCUS or LGSIL), then one of the following should occur within 6 months of the initial Pap: 1) repeat Pap smear; or 2) colposcopy.	INCLUDED BASED ON Q1 PANEL RATING
7.	Women with a Pap smear that shows ASCUS or LGSIL, and who have had the abnormality documented on at least 2 Pap smears in a 2 year period should have colposcopy performed.	7.	Women with a Pap smear that shows ASCUS or LGSIL, and who have had the abnormality documented on at least 2 Pap smears in a 2 year period should have colposcopy performed.	INCLUDED BASED ON Q1 PANEL RATING

260

Chapter 4 - Colorectal Cancer Screening

Original Indicator Proposed by Staff	Indicator Voted on by Panel	Comments/Disposition
Screening		
1. Patients documented in the chart as having one or more first degree relatives with CRC should be offered at least one of the following colon cancer screening tests beginning at age 40: • FOBT; • Sigmoidoscopy; • Colonoscopy; • DCBE.	1. Patients documented in the chart as having one or more first degree relatives with CRC should be offered at least one of the following colon cancer screening tests beginning at age 40: • **FOBT (if not done in the past 2 years);** • **Sigmoidoscopy (if not done in the past 5 years);** • **Colonoscopy (if not done in the past 10 years);** • **Double contrast barium enema (if not done in the past 5 years).**	MODIFIED: Test frequencies vary and are now specified. **ACCEPTED AS MODIFIED**
2. The chart should document discussion of the risk of CRC and risks and benefits of surveillance/screening for all patients with elevated risk of CRC due to any of the following indications: a. inflammatory bowel disease of at least 10 years duration; b. familial adenomatous polyposis syndromes; c. hereditary nonpolyposis colon cancer (HNPCC).	-- The chart should document discussion of the risk of CRC and risks and benefits of surveillance/screening for all patients with elevated risk of CRC due to any of the following indications: a. inflammatory bowel disease of at least 10 years duration; b. familial adenomatous polyposis syndromes; c. hereditary nonpolyposis colon cancer (HNPCC).	**DROPPED PRIOR TO PANEL due to feasibility concerns.**
3. Providers should offer to remove all polyps with either of the following characteristics within 6 weeks of detection: a. size greater than 1 cm; b. adenomatous histology.	2. Providers should offer to remove all polyps with either of the following characteristics within ~~6 weeks~~ **3 months** of detection: a. size greater than 1 cm; b. adenomatous histology.	MODIFIED: Panelists thought 3 months was more consistent with standard of care, especially if the referral is made from primary care. **ACCEPTED AS MODIFIED**
4. All polyps found on screening sigmoidoscopy should be biopsied at that time.	-- All polyps found on screening sigmoidoscopy should be biopsied at that time.	**DROPPED PRIOR TO PANEL.** Panelists felt that referral for biopsy was adequate.
5. Surveillance colonoscopy should not be repeated sooner than 3 years following the removal of adenomatous polyps in otherwise average risk patients.	3. Surveillance colonoscopy should not be repeated sooner than 3 years following the removal of adenomatous polyps in otherwise average risk patients.	**ACCEPTED**

Original Indicator Proposed by Staff		Indicator Voted on by Panel	Comments/Disposition
Screening			
6. Procedure note documentation for endoscopic management of polyps should include: a. whether biopsy only versus complete removal of polyps was performed; b. location of any polyps removed endoscopically; c. polyp type: sessile versus pedunculated.	4. a. b. c.	Procedure note documentation for endoscopic management of polyps should include: a. whether biopsy only versus complete removal of polyps was performed; b. location of any polyps removed endoscopically; c. polyp type: sessile versus pedunculated.	**ACCEPTED**
7. All patients with positive screening sigmoidoscopy tests should be offered a diagnostic colonoscopy.	5.	All patients with positive screening sigmoidoscopy tests should be offered a diagnostic colonoscopy **within 3 months**	MODIFIED: The time frame was specified. **ACCEPTED AS MODIFIED**
8. If a screening FOBT is positive, a diagnostic evaluation of the colon should be offered within a 6 month period.	6.	If a screening FOBT is positive, a diagnostic evaluation of the colon should be offered within a 6 **3 month** period.	MODIFIED: Panelists felt that 6 months was too long. **ACCEPTED AS MODIFIED**
9. A FOBT should be offered to those who refuse other screening tests for CRC.	--	A FOBT should be offered to those who refuse other screening tests for CRC.	**DROPPED due to low validity score.** Panelists felt that the indicator was redundant with other indicators.
10. All adults age 52 to 80 should be offered at least one of the following colon cancer screening tests: • FOBT (if not done in the past 2 years); • Sigmoidoscopy (if not done in the past 5 years); • Colonoscopy (if not done in the past 10 years); • Double contrast barium enema (if not done in the past 5 years).	7.	All **average risk** adults age 52 to 80 **50 to 80** should be offered at least one of the following colon cancer screening tests: • FOBT (if not done in the past 2 years); • Sigmoidoscopy (if not done in the past 5 years); • Colonoscopy (if not done in the past 10 years); • Double contrast barium enema (if not done in the past 5 years).	MODIFIED: Panelists wanted indicator to apply only to "average risk" patients. The age range was changed to reflect intervention age rather than age at the time of record review. **ACCEPTED AS MODIFIED**
11. Colonoscopy screening should not be done more frequently than every 5 years provided the previous colonoscopy was negative and procedure note specifies adequate exam.	8.	Colonoscopy screening should not be done in **average risk patients** more frequently than every 5 years provided the previous colonoscopy was negative and procedure note specifies adequate exam.	MODIFIED: Panelists wanted to clarify that indicator does not apply to high-risk patients, and emphasized that this indicator measures inappropriate use. **ACCEPTED AS MODIFIED**

Chapter 5 - Colorectal Cancer Treatment

	Original Indicator Proposed by Staff		Indicator Voted on by Panel	Comments/Disposition
	Staging			
1.	Patients who have undergone surgical resection for colon or rectal cancer should have documentation in the chart that colonoscopy or barium enema with sigmoidoscopy was offered within the preceding 12 months.	1.	Patients who have undergone surgical resection for colon or rectal cancer should have documentation in the chart that colonoscopy or barium enema with sigmoidoscopy was offered within the preceding 12 months.	ACCEPTED
	Treatment			
2.	Patients diagnosed with a malignant polyp should be offered a wide surgical resection within 6 weeks if any of the following are true:	2.	Patients diagnosed with a malignant polyp should be offered a wide surgical resection within 6 weeks if any of the following are true:	ACCEPTED
a.	the colonoscopy report states that the polyp was not completely excised;	a.	the colonoscopy report states that the polyp was not completely excised;	
b.	the margins are positive;	b.	the margins are positive;	
c.	lymphatic or venous invasion is present;	c.	lymphatic or venous invasion is present;	
d.	histology is grade 3 or poorly differentiated.	d.	histology is grade 3 or poorly differentiated.	
3.	Patients with a malignant polyp treated with polypectomy alone should be offered colonoscopy within 6 months of the polypectomy.	3.	Patients with a malignant polyp treated with polypectomy alone should be offered colonoscopy within 6 months of the polypectomy.	ACCEPTED
4.	Patients who are diagnosed with colon cancer and do not have metastatic disease should be offered a wide resection with anastamosis within 6 weeks of diagnosis.	4.	Patients who are diagnosed with colon cancer and do not have metastatic disease should be offered a wide resection with anastamosis within 6 weeks of diagnosis.	ACCEPTED
5.	Patients who undergo a wide surgical resection should have "negative margins" noted on the most recent final pathology report or have documentation that they were offered a repeat resection if they meet either of the following criteria:	5.	Patients who undergo a wide surgical resection should have "negative margins" noted on the most recent final pathology report or have documentation that they were offered a repeat resection if they meet either of the following criteria:	ACCEPTED
a.	Stage I colon cancer;	a.	Stage I colon cancer;	
b.	Stage II or III colon cancer that is not invading into other organs (not a T4 lesion).	b.	Stage II or III colon cancer that is not invading into other organs (not a T4 lesion).	

	Original Indicator Proposed by Staff		Indicator Voted on by Panel	Comments/Disposition
6.	Patients with Stage III colon cancer who have undergone a surgical resection should be offered adjuvant chemotherapy within 6 weeks of surgery and not before 21 days after surgery with a published 5-FU-containing regimen.	6.	Patients with Stage III colon cancer who have undergone a surgical resection should be offered adjuvant chemotherapy **to start** within 6 weeks of surgery ~~and not before 21 days after surgery~~ with a published 5-FU-containing regimen **(or be enrolled in a clinical trial with documentation of informed consent).**	MODIFIED: Panelists added an explicit clinical trial option and also felt that the minimum of 21 days after surgery was unnecessary. **ACCEPTED AS MODIFIED**
7.	Patients who are diagnosed with rectal cancer that appears clinically to be Stage I, should be offered one of the following surgical resections within 6 weeks of diagnosis: • low anterior resection; • abdominal perineal resection; • full-thickness local excision.	7.	Patients who are diagnosed **preoperatively with Stage I** rectal cancer ~~that appears clinically to be Stage I~~, should be offered one of the following surgical resections within 6 weeks of diagnosis **(or be enrolled in a clinical trial with documentation of informed consent):** • low anterior resection; • abdominal perineal resection; • full-thickness local excision.	MODIFIED: Panelists added an explicit clinical trial option and clarified other wording. **ACCEPTED AS MODIFIED**
8.	Patients who are diagnosed with rectal cancer that appears clinically to be Stage II or III, should be offered one of the following surgical resections within 6 weeks of diagnosis: • low anterior resection; • abdominal perineal resection.	8.	Patients who are diagnosed with rectal cancer that appears clinically to be Stage II or III, should be offered one of the following surgical resections within 6 weeks of diagnosis **or completion of preoperative therapy (or be enrolled in a clinical trial with documentation of informed consent):** • low anterior resection; • abdominal perineal resection.	MODIFIED: Panelists added an explicit clinical trial option and also wanted to allow time for preoperative therapy. **ACCEPTED AS MODIFIED**
9.	Patients who undergo a wide surgical resection should have "negative margins" noted on the most recent final pathology report or have documentation that they were offered a repeat resection if they meet either of the following criteria: a. Stage I rectal cancer; b. Stage II or III rectal cancer that is not invading into other organs (not a T4 lesion).	9. a. b.	Patients who undergo a wide surgical resection should have "negative margins" noted on the most recent final pathology report or have documentation that they were offered a repeat resection if they meet either of the following criteria: a. Stage I rectal cancer; b. Stage II or III rectal cancer that is not invading into other organs (not a T4 lesion).	**ACCEPTED**

	Original Indicator Proposed by Staff		Indicator Voted on by Panel	Comments/Disposition
10.	Patients with Stage II and III rectal cancer (defined pathologically) who undergo surgical resection should be offered one of the following treatments (*this indicator only applies to patients who have had a surgical resection*): • postoperative radiation therapy of 45-55 Gy to the pelvis with chemotherapy containing 5-FU to begin not sooner than 4 weeks after surgery and not more than 12 weeks after surgery; • preoperative radiation therapy to the pelvis to begin not more than 6 weeks after diagnosis; • preoperative radiation therapy with chemotherapy containing 5-FU to begin not more than 6 weeks after diagnosis.	10.	Patients with Stage II and III rectal cancer (defined pathologically) who undergo surgical resection should be offered one of the following treatments **(or be enrolled in a clinical trial with documentation of informed consent)** (*this indicator only applies to patients who have had a surgical resection*): • postoperative radiation therapy of 45-55 Gy to the pelvis with chemotherapy containing 5-FU to begin not sooner than 4 weeks after surgery and not more than 12 weeks after surgery; • preoperative radiation therapy to the pelvis to begin not more than 6 weeks after diagnosis **and discussion of postoperative therapy;** • preoperative radiation therapy with chemotherapy containing 5-FU to begin not more than 6 weeks after diagnosis **and discussion of postoperative therapy.**	MODIFIED: Panelists added an explicit clinical trial option and thought that post-operative chemotherapy should always be discussed. **ACCEPTED AS MODIFIED**
11.	Patients receiving 5-FU chemotherapy should have a CBC checked not more than 48 hours prior to the first dose in each cycle.	--	Patients receiving 5-FU chemotherapy should have a CBC checked not more than 48 hours prior to the first dose in each cycle.	**DROPPED due to low validity score.**
12.	Patients should not receive 5-FU chemotherapy if any of the following are documented in the two days prior to initiation of therapy: a. WBC < 2,000 or ANC < 1,500; b. stomatitis that prevents them from eating; c. severe diarrhea (seven or more stools a day).	--	Patients should not receive 5-FU chemotherapy if any of the following are documented in the two days prior to initiation of therapy: a. WBC < 2,000 or ANC < 1,500; b. stomatitis that prevents them from eating; c. severe diarrhea (seven or more stools a day).	**DROPPED due to low validity score.**
13.	Patients with Stages I, II, and III colorectal cancer should receive a visit with a physician for a history and physical where colorectal cancer is addressed in the assessment and plan at least every 6 months for 3 years after initial treatment.	--	Patients with Stages I, II, and III colorectal cancer should receive a visit with a physician for a history and physical where colorectal cancer is addressed in the assessment and plan at least every 6 months for 3 years after **initial initiation of** treatment.	**DROPPED due to low validity score.**

265

Original Indicator Proposed by Staff		Indicator Voted on by Panel	Comments/Disposition
	11. (16)	Patients with ~~Stage IV~~ metastatic colon cancer should have ~~chemotherapeutic~~ options discussed within three weeks of staging **(or be enrolled in a clinical trial with documentation of informed consent).**	**PROPOSED AND ACCEPTED BY Q2 PANEL.** Explicit clinical trial option added.
Follow-up			
	12.	Patients with Stages I, II, and III colorectal cancer should receive colonoscopy or double contrast barium enema within a year of curative surgery if it did not occur within 12 months preoperatively.	**ACCEPTED**
14. Patients with Stages I, II, and III colorectal cancer should receive colonoscopy or double contrast barium enema within a year of curative surgery if it did not occur within 12 months preoperatively.			
	13.	Patients with Stages I, II, and III colorectal cancer should receive colonoscopy or double contrast barium enema ~~three years~~ **within one year** after surgery and, **if normal, at least** every five years thereafter.	**MODIFIED:** Panelists shortened time frame and clarified that follow-up time frame is for normal results. **ACCEPTED AS MODIFIED**
15. Patients with Stages I, II, and III colorectal cancer should receive colonoscopy or double contrast barium enema three years after surgery and every five years thereafter.			

266

	Original Indicator Proposed by Staff		Indicator Voted on by Panel	Comments/Disposition
	Screening and Prevention			
1.	HIV+ patients should be offered PCP prophylaxis within one month of meeting any of the following conditions:	1.	HIV+ patients should be offered PCP prophylaxis within one month of meeting any of the following conditions:	**"a, c" ACCEPTED** "b" DROPPED due to low validity score. Thrush was only considered to be associated with, and not a predictor of, PCP. Panelists noted that the more recent recommendations for prophylaxis do not include thrush. "d" PROPOSED AND ACCEPTED BY Q2 PANEL. CD4 percentage is also used in practice.
	a. CD4 count dropping below 200;	a.	CD4 count dropping below 200;	
	b. thrush;	-- b.	thrush;	
	c. completion of active treatment of PCP.	c.	completion of active treatment of PCP;	
			d. CD4 below 15%.	
2.	HIV+ patients who do not have active TB and who have not previously received TB prophylaxis should be offered TB prophylaxis within one month of meeting any of following conditions:	2.	HIV+ patients who do not have active TB and who have not **ever** previously received TB prophylaxis should be offered TB prophylaxis within one month of meeting any of the following conditions:	MODIFIED: Clarified wording.
	a. current PPD > 5 mm;	a.	current PPD > 5 mm;	
	b. provider noting that patient has had PPD > 5 mm administered at anytime since HIV diagnosis;	b.	provider noting that patient has had PPD > 5 mm administered at anytime since HIV diagnosis;	**"a, b" ACCEPTED AS MODIFIED** **"c" DROPPED due to disagreement in validity.** Panelists felt that contact information may not be readily available except from the health department.
	c. contact with person with active TB.	--	contact with person with active TB.	
3.	HIV+ patients who do not have active toxoplasmosis should be offered toxoplasmosis prophylaxis within one month of meeting all of the following conditions:	3.	HIV+ patients who do not have active toxoplasmosis should be offered toxoplasmosis prophylaxis within one month of meeting **either of the** following conditions:	MODIFIED: Typographical error corrected. **ACCEPTED AS MODIFIED**
	• Toxo IgG positive;		• Toxo IgG positive **and CD4 count dropping below 100;**	
	• CD4 count dropping below 100		• CD4 count dropping below 100	
	• Completion of therapy for active toxoplasmosis.		• Completion of therapy for active toxoplasmosis.	
4.	Toxoplasmosis serology should be offered within one month of initial diagnosis of HIV.	4.	HIV+ **patients should have** toxoplasmosis serology **documented** should be offered within one month of initial diagnosis of HIV.	MODIFIED: Panelists simplified the indicator to broaden the eligible population to all people with HIV and improve the feasibility in finding information on toxoplasmosis. **ACCEPTED AS MODIFIED**
5.	HIV+ patients should be offered MAC prophylaxis within one month of a CD4 count dropping below 50.	5.	HIV+ patients should be offered MAC prophylaxis within one month of a CD4 count dropping below 50.	**ACCEPTED**

267

Original Indicator Proposed by Staff		Indicator Voted on by Panel	Comments/Disposition
Screening and Prevention			
6.	HIV+ patients should have a documented pneumovax.	6.	HIV+ patients **with a lowest recorded CD4 count > 200** should have a documented pneumovax.	MODIFIED: Panelists felt that pneumovax should not be offered to those with a CD4 count below 200 because of impaired vaccine response. **ACCEPTED AS MODIFIED**
7.	HIV+ patients with a lowest recorded CD4 count of less than 100 should have had a fundoscopic exam in the past year.	7.	HIV+ patients with a lowest recorded CD4 count of less than 100 should have had a **yearly dilated** fundoscopic exam ~~in the past year~~.	MODIFIED: Panelists added "dilated" to ensure an adequate exam. **ACCEPTED AS MODIFIED**
8.	VDRL or RPR should be offered within one month of initial diagnosis of HIV infection unless done in past year.	8.	**HIV+ patients should have a VDRL or RPR documented in the chart.** ~~should be offered within one month of initial diagnosis of HIV infection unless done in past year.~~	MODIFIED: Panelists simplified the indicator to broaden the eligible population to all people with HIV and improve the feasibility of finding information on VDRL or RPR. **ACCEPTED AS MODIFIED**
		--	Sexually active HIV+ patients should be offered a VDRL/RPR annually.	**DROPPED due to low validity score.** Panelists felt this indicator was redundant with the modified indicator 8. They also questioned whether there would be information on sexual activity in the charts.
9.	Sexually active HIV+ patients should be offered a VDRL/RPR annually.			
Diagnosis			
10.	The following tests should be obtained within one month of initial diagnosis of HIV infection: a. CBC; b. HIV RNA (viral load); c. CD4.	9. a. b. c.	The following tests should be obtained within one month of initial diagnosis of HIV infection: a. CBC; b. HIV RNA (viral load); c. CD4.	**ACCEPTED**
11.	HIV+ patients with CD4 counts > 500 should be offered the following tests within 6 months: a. CD4; b. viral loads.	10. a. b.	HIV+ patients with CD4 counts > ~~500~~ **300** should be offered the following tests **every** 6 months: a. **CD4** count or percentage; b. ~~viral loads~~ **HIV RNA (viral load)**.	MODIFIED: Panelists lowered the CD4 threshold because patients with more impaired immune function need closer follow-up. They also clarified test terminology. **ACCEPTED AS MODIFIED**

268

Original Indicator Proposed by Staff		Indicator Voted on by Panel	Comments/Disposition
12	HIV+ patients with CD4 counts < 500 should be offered the following tests within 3 months: a. CD4; b. viral loads.	11. HIV+ patients with ~~CD4 counts < 500~~ **detectable viral loads** should be offered the following tests within ~~4~~ 3 months: -- a. CD4 **count or percentage**; a. b. ~~viral loads~~ **HIV RNA (viral load)**.	MODIFIED: Panelists felt that 3 months was too short and clarified test terminology. Panelists indicated that patients with any detectable viral load should be monitored. "a" **DROPPED due to low validity score.** **ACCEPTED AS MODIFIED**
13	HIV+ patients on antiretroviral therapy should have been offered the following tests within the past 3 months: a. CD4; b. viral load; c. CBC.	12. HIV+ patients on antiretroviral therapy have been offered the following tests within the past ~~3~~ 4 months: a. CD4 **count or percentage**; b. **HIV RNA** (viral load); c. CBC.	MODIFIED: Panelists compromised on a 4-month time period and clarified test terminology. **ACCEPTED AS MODIFIED**
	Treatment		
14	HIV+ patients should receive adequate antiretroviral treatment within one month of any of the following conditions being met: a. CD4 > 500 and viral load >30k; b. CD4 350-500 and viral load >10k; c. CD4 <350; d. any AIDS-defining condition; e. thrush.	13. HIV+ patients should receive adequate antiretroviral treatment within one month of any of the following conditions being met **(or be enrolled in a clinical trial with documentation of informed consent)**: a. CD4 >= 500 and viral load >30k; b. CD4 350- ~~500~~ 499 and viral load >10k; c. CD4 <350; d. any AIDS-defining condition; e. thrush.	MODIFIED: Panelists added an explicit clinical trial option and clarified the CD4 cutoffs. **ACCEPTED AS MODIFIED**
15	Protease inhibitors should not be prescribed concurrently with astemizole, terfenadine, rifampin or cisapride.	14. Protease inhibitors should not be prescribed concurrently with astemizole, terfenadine, rifampin or cisapride.	**ACCEPTED**
		15. (18) HIV+ patients should be counseled regarding high risk behavior: a. at the time of HIV diagnosis; b. within one month of presentation with an initial infection of STD.	**PROPOSED AND ACCEPTED BY Q2 PANEL-** Panelists felt that education is critical to prevent HIV/STD transmission.

Original Indicator Proposed by Staff		Indicator Voted on by Panel	Comments/Disposition
Follow-up			
16.	HIV+ patients should be offered viral load measurement within one month of initiation or change in antiretroviral treatment.	16.	HIV+ patients should be offered viral load measurement within ~~one month~~ two months of initiation or change in antiretroviral treatment.	MODIFIED: Panelists felt one month was too short. **ACCEPTED AS MODIFIED**
		17. (17)	**HIV+ patients started on protease inhibitors should have documented counseling regarding compliance with therapy within 1 month of the start of therapy.**	**PROPOSED AND ACCEPTED BY Q2 PANEL.** Compliance is critical to effective treatment and to prevent resistant strains of HIV.

270

Chapter 7 - Lung Cancer

	Original Indicator Proposed by Staff		Indicator Voted on by Panel	Comments/Disposition
	Diagnosis			
1.	Patients without a prior diagnosis of cancer (except non-melanoma skin cancer) with a mass (>= 3 cm) on chest x-ray or CT scan of the chest should have one of the following diagnostic endpoints documented in the chart within 2 months of the radiological study: • Chest CT with multiple nodules; • Sputum cytology diagnostic of cancer (expectorated or bronchoscopic washing); • Cytology report from a fine needle aspiration of the mass; • Pathology report from lymph node biopsy that is diagnostic of cancer; • Pathology report from lung biopsy; • Operative report indicating surgical resection of the mass.	1.	Patients without a prior diagnosis of **metastatic** cancer (except non-melanoma skin cancer) with a **solitary** mass (>= 3 cm) on chest x-ray or CT scan of the chest should have one of the following diagnostic endpoints **a tissue or cytologic diagnosis of pathologic process** documented in the chart within 2 months of the radiological study **unless contraindicated.** • Chest CT with multiple nodules; • Sputum cytology diagnostic of cancer (expectorated or bronchoscopic washing); • Cytology report from a fine needle aspiration of the mass; • Pathology report from lymph node biopsy that is diagnostic of cancer; • Pathology report from lung biopsy; • Operative report indicating surgical resection of the mass.	MODIFIED: Panelists wanted to consolidate the description of a histological diagnosis and simplify the wording for operationalization. **ACCEPTED AS MODIFIED**

271

Original Indicator Proposed by Staff		Indicator Voted on by Panel	Comments/Disposition
Diagnosis			
2. Patients without a prior diagnosis of cancer (except non-melanoma skin cancer) with a solitary nodule (< 3 cm) on chest x-ray or CT scan of the chest should have one of the following diagnostic endpoints documented in the chart within 2 months of the radiological study: • Report of chest x-ray or CT scan of the chest from at least 2 years prior to the index study which shows a nodule of the same size in the same location; • Chest x-ray or CT scan report describes the nodule has having central, diffuse, speckled, or laminar calcifications; • Chest CT scan report states that the density of the nodule is > 160 Hounsfield units; • Chest CT with multiple nodules; • Sputum cytology, bronchoscopic washing, or bronchoscopic brushing diagnostic of cancer • Cytology report from a fine needle aspiration of the mass; • Pathology report from lymph node biopsy that is diagnostic of cancer; • Pathology report from biopsy of nodule; • Operative report indicating surgical resection of the mass.	2.	Patients without a prior diagnosis of cancer (except non-melanoma skin cancer) with a solitary nodule (< 3 cm) on chest x-ray or CT scan of the chest should have one of the following ~~diagnostic endpoints~~ documented in the chart within 2 months of the radiological study: • Report of chest x-ray or CT scan of the chest from at least 2 years prior to the index study which shows a nodule of the same size in the same location; • Chest x-ray or CT scan report describes the nodule has having central, diffuse, speckled, or laminar calcifications; • Chest CT scan report states that the density of the nodule is > 160 Hounsfield units; • Chest CT with multiple nodules; • Sputum cytology, bronchoscopic washing, or bronchoscopic brushing diagnostic of cancer; • Cytology report from a fine needle aspiration of the mass; • Pathology report from lymph node biopsy that is diagnostic of cancer; • Pathology report from biopsy of nodule; • Operative report indicating surgical resection of the mass.	MODIFIED: Wording clarified. **ACCEPTED AS MODIFIED**

272

	Original Indicator Proposed by Staff		Indicator Voted on by Panel	Comments/Disposition
	Treatment			
3.	Patients with non-small cell lung cancer should have both of the following not more than 3 months prior to lung resection: a. pulmonary function assessment with either pulmonary function tests (FEV1, maximum ventilatory volume < 50% on pulmonary function tests; b. EKG.	3. a. b.	Patients with non-small cell lung cancer should have both of the following not more than 3 months prior to lung resection: a. pulmonary function assessment with either pulmonary function tests (FEV1, maximum ventilatory volume) or a quantitative ventilation scan or a quantitative perfusion scan; b. EKG.	ACCEPTED.
4.	Patients with Stage I and II non-small cell lung cancer should be offered a lung resection (pneumonectomy, lobectomy, or wedge resection) within 6 weeks of diagnosis unless any of the following are documented: a. another metastatic cancer; b. FEV1 < 40% on pulmonary function tests; c. maximum ventilatory volume < 50% on pulmonary function tests; d. pCO$_2$ > 45 mm Hg on an arterial blood gas; e. <=0.8 liter perfusion to contralateral lung by quantitative perfusion scan; f. documentation in chart that patient is medically "unacceptable risk" for surgery.	4. -- -- -- -- -- --	Patients with Stage I and II non-small cell lung cancer should be offered a lung resection (pneumonectomy, lobectomy, or wedge resection) within 6 weeks of diagnosis unless **contraindicated**. ~~any of the following are documented:~~ a. ~~another metastatic cancer;~~ b. ~~FEV1 < 40% on pulmonary function tests;~~ c. ~~maximum ventilatory volume < 50% on pulmonary function tests;~~ d. ~~pCO$_2$ > 45 mm Hg on an arterial blood gas;~~ e. ~~<=0.8 liter perfusion to contralateral lung by quantitative perfusion scan;~~ f. ~~documentation in chart that patient is medically "unacceptable risk" for surgery.~~	MODIFIED: The term "contraindicated" will be defined during operationalization rather than listing all of the contraindication as part of the indicator. ACCEPTED AS MODIFIED
5.	Patients with Stage I or II non-small cell lung cancer who do not undergo a lung resection should be offered radiation therapy to the chest (>= 5000 cGy) within 6 weeks of diagnosis.	5.	Patients with Stage I or II non-small cell lung cancer who do not undergo a lung resection should be offered radiation therapy to the chest (>= 5000 cGy) within 6 weeks of diagnosis.	ACCEPTED

273

	Original Indicator Proposed by Staff		Indicator Voted on by Panel	Comments/Disposition
	Treatment			
6.	Patients with Stage III non-small cell lung cancer with good performance status should be offered at least one of the following within 6 weeks of diagnosis: • thoracotomy with surgical resection of the tumor; • radiation therapy to the thorax; • chemotherapy.	6.	Patients with Stage III non-small cell lung cancer with good performance status should be offered at least one of the following within 6 weeks of diagnosis (**unless contraindicated or enrolled in a clinical trial with documentation of informed consent**): • thoracotomy with surgical resection of the tumor; • radiation therapy to the thorax with chemotherapy. • ~~chemotherapy.~~	MODIFIED: An explicit clinical trial option was added. Panelists felt that there was no consensus on the effectiveness of chemotherapy alone. **ACCEPTED AS MODIFIED**
7.	Patients with Stage IV non-small cell lung cancer and good performance status should be offered chemotherapy within 6 weeks of diagnosis.	7.	Patients with Stage IV non-small cell lung cancer and good performance status should **have be** offered chemotherapy **discussed within 6 weeks** of diagnosis (**or be enrolled in a clinical trial with documentation of informed consent**).	MODIFIED: An explicit clinical trial option was added. Panelists preferred the term "discussed" as both chemotherapy and its contraindications should be considered. **ACCEPTED AS MODIFIED**
8.	Patients with non-small cell lung cancer who have metastases on MRI or CT of the brain should be offered one of the following treatments within 2 weeks of the MRI or CT: • radiation therapy to the brain; • surgical resection of the metastasis; • stereotactic radiosurgery.	8.	Patients with non-small cell lung cancer who have **first** metastases on MRI or CT of the brain should be offered one of the following treatments within **≥ 1** week of the MRI or CT (**or be enrolled in a clinical trial with documentation of informed consent**): • radiation therapy to the brain; • surgical resection of the metastasis; • stereotactic radiosurgery.	MODIFIED: An explicit clinical trial option was added. Panelists also clarified criteria ("first" added" and felt that the 2 week time frame was too long. **ACCEPTED AS MODIFIED**
9.	Patients with limited small cell lung cancer should be offered combined modality therapy with radiation therapy (>= 5,000 cGy) and chemotherapy within 6 weeks of diagnosis.	9.	Patients with limited small cell lung cancer should be offered combined modality therapy with radiation therapy (>= 5,000 cGy) and chemotherapy within **≥ 2** weeks of diagnosis (**or be enrolled in a clinical trial with documentation of informed consent**).	MODIFIED: An explicit clinical trial option was added. Panelists felt that 6 weeks was too long. **ACCEPTED AS MODIFIED**
10.	Patients with extensive small cell lung cancer should be offered chemotherapy within 6 weeks of diagnosis.	10.	Patients with extensive small cell lung cancer should be offered chemotherapy within **≥ 2** weeks of diagnosis.	MODIFIED: Panelists felt that 6 weeks was too long. **ACCEPTED AS MODIFIED**

Original Indicator Proposed by Staff		Indicator Voted on by Panel		Comments/Disposition
Treatment				
11.	Patients with small cell lung cancer who have metastases on MRI or CT of the brain should be offered either of the following within 2 weeks of diagnosis of brain metastases (unless they have received both previously): • chemotherapy; • radiation therapy to the brain.	11.	Patients with small cell lung cancer who have **first** metastases on MRI or CT of the brain should be offered either of the following within 2 **1 week** of diagnosis of brain metastases (unless they have received both previously): • chemotherapy; • radiation therapy to the brain.	**MODIFIED:** Panelists felt that 2 weeks was too long and clarified criteria ("first" added). ACCEPTED AS MODIFIED
12.	Patients with small cell lung cancer who have bone pain and a corresponding positive radiographic study should be offered either of the following within 3 weeks of presenting with the complaint of pain (unless they have received both previously): • chemotherapy; • radiation therapy to the region.	--	Patients with small cell lung cancer who have bone pain and a corresponding positive radiographic study should be offered either of the following within 3 weeks **1 week** of presenting with the complaint of pain (unless they have received both previously): • chemotherapy; • radiation therapy to the region.	**DROPPED due to low validity score.** Panelists felt that pain was an important indication for treatment, but had concerns about clinical heterogeneity of the eligible population.

275

Chapter 9 - Prostate Cancer Treatment

	Original Indicator Proposed by Staff		Indicator Voted on by Panel	Comments/Disposition
	Diagnosis			
1.	A patient *without* any previously known diagnosis of cancer who has an x-ray or radionuclide bone scan with blastic or lytic lesions, or with a notation that the findings are consistent with metastases, should be offered all of the following within the 12 months prior or the 3 weeks following the date of the x-ray or bone scan: a. digital rectal exam; b. PSA.	--	A ~~patient~~ **Men** *without* any previously known diagnosis of cancer who ~~has~~ **have** an x-ray or radionuclide bone scan with blastic or lytic lesions, or with a notation that the findings are consistent with metastases, should be offered all **both** of the following within the 12 months prior **to** or the 3 weeks following the date of the x-ray or bone scan: a. digital rectal exam; b. PSA.	**DROPPED due to low validity score.**
2.	Patients with a new diagnosis of prostate cancer, who have not had a serum PSA in the prior three months, should have serum PSA checked within one month after diagnosis or prior to any treatment, whichever comes first.	1.	~~Patients~~ **Men** with a new diagnosis of prostate cancer, who have not had a serum PSA in the prior three months, should have serum PSA checked within one month after diagnosis or prior to any treatment, whichever comes first.	MODIFIED: Wording clarified. **ACCEPTED AS MODIFIED**
3.	Patients with a new diagnosis of prostate cancer who have a PSA > 10mg/ml should be offered a radionuclide bone scan within 1 month or prior to initiation of any treatment, whichever is first.	2.	~~Patients~~ **Men** with a new diagnosis of prostate cancer who have a PSA > 10mg/ml should be offered a radionuclide bone scan within 1 month or prior to initiation of any treatment, whichever is **comes** first.	MODIFIED: Wording clarified. **ACCEPTED AS MODIFIED**
	Treatment			
4.	Men over 60 with minimal prostate cancer (Stage 0/A1) should not be offered any of the following treatments: a. bilateral orchiectomy; b. LHRH analogue ; c. antiandrogen; d. radical prostatectomy; e. radiation therapy.	3. a. b. c. -- --	Men over 60 with minimal prostate cancer (Stage 0/A1) should not be offered any of the following treatments: a. bilateral orchiectomy; b. LHRH analogue; c. antiandrogen; d. radical prostatectomy; e. radiation therapy.	"a", "b", "c" ACCEPTED "d, e" DROPPED due to disagreement on validity.

Original Indicator Proposed by Staff		Indicator Voted on by Panel	Comments/Disposition
	4. (4)	Men over 60 with minimal prostate cancer (Stage T1C with Gleason <= 4 and PSA <= 10) should not be offered any of the following treatments: a. bilateral orchiectomy; b. LHRH analogue; c. antiandrogen.	**Panelists considered and ACCEPTED indicator with modified stage and grade (for "a, b, c" only).** Panelists indicated that T1C diagnoses are made more often now.
5. Men under 65, who do not have coronary artery disease or a second cancer should be offered radical prostatectomy or radiation therapy for localized prostate cancer (Stage I & II/A2 & B) within 3 months of staging.	5.	Men under age 65 with localized prostate cancer (Stage I or II/A2 or B) and a Gleason score <= 6 should have all of the following treatment options discussed within 3 months of diagnosis (unless contraindicated or enrolled in a clinical trial with documentation of informed consent): • Radiation therapy; • Prostatectomy; • Watchful waiting.	MODIFIED: Panelists reworded the indicator to include a Gleason score and an explicit clinical trial option. Panelists also felt that watchful waiting was appropriate care, and that "offered" should be changed to "discussed" in order to account for patients who may have a limited life expectancy. **ACCEPTED AS MODIFIED**
6. Men with metastatic prostate cancer (Stage IV/D) should be offered at least one of the following androgen blockade treatments within three months of staging: • bilateral orchiectomy; • LHRH analogue; • Antiandrogen.	6.	Men with metastatic prostate cancer (Stage IV/D) should be offered at least one of the following androgen blockade treatments within three months of staging: • bilateral orchiectomy; • LHRH analogue **with or without antiandrogen.** • ~~antiandrogen~~	MODIFIED: Panelists felt that antiandrogen alone is not adequate therapy. **ACCEPTED AS MODIFIED**
7. Men who undergo orchiectomy for the treatment of prostate cancer should have documented that they were offered treatment with an LHRH analogue or antiandrogen within 12 months prior to surgery.	7.	Men who undergo orchiectomy for the treatment of prostate cancer should have documented that they were offered treatment with an LHRH analogue **(with or without antiandrogen)** ~~or antiandrogen~~ within 12 months prior to surgery.	MODIFIED: Panelists felt that antiandrogen alone is not adequate therapy. **ACCEPTED AS MODIFIED**

	Original Indicator Proposed by Staff		Indicator Voted on by Panel	Comments/Disposition
8.	Prostate cancer patients who present with acute low back pain should have documentation within 24 hours of the complaint or in the preceding 3 months of one of the following: • a CT scan of the spine *without* blastic or lytic lesions or compression fractures; • a CT myelogram; • an MRI of the spine.	8.	**Metastatic** prostate cancer patients who present with acute low back pain **with radiculopathy** should have documentation within 24 hours of the complaint or in the preceding 3 months of **presentation of** one of the following: • a CT scan of the spine *without* blastic or lytic lesions or compression fractures; • a CT myelogram; • an MRI of the spine.	MODIFIED: Panelists wanted to restrict back pain more to that which may be due to spinal cord compression. They also narrowed the time frame and clarified that the indicator only applies to metastatic cases. **ACCEPTED AS MODIFIED**
9.	Prostate cancer patients with evidence of cord compression on MRI scan of the spine or CT myelogram should be offered one of the following within 24 hours of the radiologic study: • radiation therapy to the spine at a total dose between 3000 cGy and 4500 cGy over 2-4 weeks; • decompressive laminectomy.	9.	Prostate cancer patients with evidence of cord compression **from tumor** on MRI scan of the spine or CT myelogram should be offered one of the following within 24 hours of the radiologic study: • radiation therapy to the spine at a total dose between 3000 cGy and 4500 cGy over 2-4 weeks; • decompressive laminectomy.	MODIFIED: Wording clarified. **ACCEPTED AS MODIFIED**
10.	Prostate cancer patients with evidence of cord compression on MRI scan of the spine or CT myelogram should be offered at least 4 mg dexamethazone IV prior to the radiologic study or within 1 hour of its completion, followed by dexamethasone 4 mg IV or PO q six hours for at least 72 hours.	10.	Prostate cancer patients with evidence of cord compression **from tumor** on MRI scan of the spine or CT myelogram should be offered at least 4 mg dexamethazone IV prior to the radiologic study or within ± 4 hours of its completion, followed by dexamethasone 4 mg IV or PO six hours for at least 72 hours.	MODIFIED: Panelists felt that dexamethazone within one hour of completion of study was too narrow a time frame. **ACCEPTED AS MODIFIED**
		11. (11)	Men under age 75 with localized prostate cancer (Stage I or II/A2 or B) and a Gleason score >= 7 should be offered both of the following treatment options within 3 months of diagnosis (unless contraindicated or enrolled in a clinical trial with documentation of informed consent): • radiation therapy; • radical prostatectomy.	PROPOSED AND ACCEPTED BY Q2 PANEL
		12. (12) a. b. c. d.	Men with prostate cancer who present with acute back pain should have the presence or absence of all the following elicited on the day of presentation: a. **bladder dysfunction;** b. **bowel dysfunction;** c. **weakness or radicular symptoms;** d. **sensory loss.**	PROPOSED AND ACCEPTED BY Q2 PANEL

278

Chapter 10 - Skin Cancer Screening

	Original Indicator Proposed by Staff		Indicator Voted on by Panel	Comments/Disposition
	Primary Prevention			
1.	When a patient is noted to have a sunburn, the chart should document counseling regarding avoidance of midday sun, use of protective clothing, and/or use of sunscreens.	--	When a patient is noted to have a sunburn, the chart should document counseling regarding avoidance of midday sun, use of protective clothing, and/or use of sunscreens.	**DROPPED due to low feasibility score.**
2.	Patients who have evidence of aktinic keratosis or solar keratosis (AK), should be counseled regarding avoidance of midday sun, use of protective clothing, and/or use of sunscreens within 1 year before or after diagnosis.	1.	Patients who have evidence of aktinic keratosis or solar keratosis (AK), should be counseled regarding avoidance of midday sun, use of protective clothing, and/or use of sunscreens within 1 year before or after diagnosis.	**ACCEPTED**
3.	All patients noted to have strong skin cancer risk factors should be instructed in midday sun avoidance, use of protective clothing, and/or use of sunscreens within 1 year before or after note of high risk.	--	All patients noted to have strong skin cancer risk factors should be instructed in midday sun avoidance, use of protective clothing, and/or use of sunscreens within 1 year before or after note of high risk.	**DROPPED due to low feasibility score.** Panelists felt that risk factors may not be documented and that that would not necessarily reflect poor quality.
	Secondary Prevention/Skin Self-exam			
4.	All patients noted to have strong skin cancer risk factors should be instructed in skin self-examination within 1 year before or after note of high risk.	--	All patients noted to have strong skin cancer risk factors should be instructed in skin self-examination within 1 year before or after note of high risk.	**DROPPED due to low validity score.** Evidence linking examination with improved outcomes is lacking.
5.	All patients with a personal history of melanoma or non-melanoma skin cancer (NMSC) should be counseled to do skin self-examination within 1 year before or after the history is documented.	2.	All patients with a personal history of melanoma or ~~non-melanoma skin cancer (NMSC)~~ should be counseled to do skin self-examination within 1 year before or after the history is documented.	MODIFIED: Panelists felt that this was not critical for those with NMSC because NMSC causes less morbidity/mortality. **ACCEPTED AS MODIFIED**
	Secondary Prevention/ Clinician Screening			
6.	Patients diagnosed with NMSC or multiple AKs in the past 5 years should have a skin exam documented in the past 12 months.	3.	Patients **with a history of** ~~diagnosed with NMSC~~ or multiple AKs in the past 5 years should have a skin exam documented in the past 12 months.	MODIFIED **ACCEPTED AS MODIFIED**
7.	Referral to a dermatologist for surveillance/screening should be documented if a patient has either of the following: a. personal history of cutaneous melanoma (CM); b. multiple common or atypical moles plus a family history of CM (possible FAM-M phenotype).	--	Referral to a dermatologist for surveillance/screening should be documented if a patient has either of the following: a. personal history of cutaneous melanoma (CM); b. multiple common or atypical moles plus a family history of CM (possible FAM-M phenotype).	**DROPPED PRIOR TO PANEL.** Panelists indicated that it was difficult to identify dermatologists from the medical record alone.

	Original Indicator Proposed by Staff		Indicator Voted on by Panel	Comments/Disposition
8.	All patients newly diagnosed with melanoma should be advised to have family members undergo a screening skin exam.	--	All patients newly diagnosed with melanoma should be advised to have family members undergo a screening skin exam.	**DROPPED due to low validity score.** Evidence linking screening to improved outcomes is poor.
9.	All patients with a documented family history of melanoma in a first degree relative should have a screening skin exam at least once in the year preceding or subsequent to documentation.	--	All patients with a documented family history of melanoma in a first degree relative should have a screening skin exam at least once in the year preceding or subsequent to documentation.	DROPPED due to low validity score. **Panelists did not feel that a family history of melanoma was a sufficient reason to require a skin exam.**
		4. (9)	**All patients with a documented personal history of melanoma should have a screening skin exam at least once in the year preceding or subsequent to documentation.**	**Panelists considered and ACCEPTED an indicator for personal history.** Panelists felt that a personal history of melanoma was a sufficient reason to require a skin exam.

280

Chapter 11 - Cancer Pain and Palliation

Original Indicator Proposed by Staff		Indicator Voted on by Panel	Comments/Disposition
Diagnosis			
	1. (1)	Patients with metastatic cancer to bone should have the presence or absence of pain noted at least every 6 months.	PROPOSED AND ACCEPTED BY Q2 PANEL
Treatment			
	2. (2)	Cancer patients whose pain is uncontrolled should be offered a change in pain management within 24 hours of the pain complaint.	PROPOSED AND ACCEPTED BY Q2 PANEL
	-- (3)	Patients with painful bony metastases, who are noted to be unresponsive to or intolerant of narcotic analgesia, should be offered one of the following within one week of the notation of pain: • radiation therapy to the sites of pain; • radioactive strontium therapy.	PROPOSED BUT DROPPED BY Q2 PANEL due to low validity score.
	3. (4)	Patients receiving emetogenic chemotherapy should be offered concurrent potent antiemetic therapy (e.g. 5HT blockade).	PROPOSED AND ACCEPTED BY Q2 PANEL